Case Studies in
Clinical Examination

Owen Epstein MBBCh FRCP
Consultant Physician and Gastroenterologist
Clinical Tutor and Director of the Endoscopy Unit
Royal Free Hospital NHS Trust
London, UK

G David Perkin BA MB FRCP
Consultant Neurologist
Charing Cross Hospital and Hillingdon Hospital
London, UK

David P de Bono MA MD FRCP
British Heart Foundation Professor of Cardiology (University of Leicester)
Glenfield General Hospital, Leicester
Honorary Consultant Cardiologist
Groby Road General Hospital
Leicester, UK

John Cookson MD FRCP
Consultant Physician and Clinical Tutor
Department of Respiratory Medicine
Glenfield General Hospital
Leicester, UK

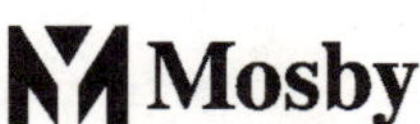

London Baltimore Barcelona Bogotá Boston Buenos Aires Caracas Carlsbad, CA Chicago Madrid Mexico City Milan Naples, FL New York Philadelphia St. Louis Seoul Singapore Sydney Taipei Tokyo Toronto Wiesbaden

Project Manager:	Tuan Hô
Publisher's Assistant:	Laura Parker
Designer:	Lara Last
Production:	Siobhan Egan
Index:	Anne McCarthy
Publisher:	Richard Furn

CONTENTS

• The page and chapter numbers cited at the top of each answer page refer to Epstein *et al.*, *Clinical Examination* (Mosby, 1992)

IT is important to remember that the practice of medidcine remains focused around history and examination. Despite enormous technological leaps in the past decades, most clinical problems can be resolved by taking a good history and eliciting physical signs.

Indeed, for the foreseeable future, clinical examination will remain at the very centre of medical practice. The 52 case histories in this book are a companion to the *Clinical Examination* textbook, to which each case is cross-referenced. Each case has been presented to emphasize the importance of history and examination in the problem-solving exercise, and should provide a stimulus for further reading.

I am indebted to Dr Bruce MacFarlane and Dr Harriet Gordon who made a considerable contribution to the format of this book. I am sure that you will be both informed and entertained by the diverse spectrum of clinical scenarios which we have compiled.

Owen Epstein

CASE 1

Alan Goodman, a 57-year-old lawyer, reports that the previous Friday he and his wife celebrated their wedding anniversary by dining at a local restaurant, where they shared a Chateaubriand. The evening was interrupted by "the food sticking in my chest", causing intense discomfort. His wife thought he was having a heart attack (he smoked ten cigars a day, despite her admonitions). He had then vomited out a plug of semi-chewed food, with relief of his pain. On further enquiry, he reports a sticking sensation with certain foods over the past year. This was easily overcome by drinking water with his meals, which he claims also cleared up the heartburn which had plagued him all his life.

QUESTIONS

1. What is a typical history for gastro-oesophageal reflux disease (GORD)?

2. What complication has occurred in this patient?

3. Give a differential diagnosis for the dysphagia in this patient, and discuss how the presenting problem of dysphagia may vary from condition to condition

NOTES FOR REVISION

YOUR ANSWERS

1 Typical history for GORD

2 Complication occurring in Mr Goodman

3 Differential diagnosis for dysphagia in Mr Goodman, and how the presenting problem of dysphagia may vary from condition to condition

ANSWERS

1. GORD is a diagnosis made on history and confirmed with endoscopy. The patient may be overweight (the increase in intra-abdominal pressure promoting reflux) but obesity and GORD are not inevitably associated. A typical history is that of burning epigastric pain, radiating retrosternally. This may be associated with a bitter/acidic taste in the mouth and/or a 'water brash', from reflex salivation. The pain may have clear dietary precipitants, be aggravated by bending over/lying down, be rapidly relieved with antacids and ameliorated by inhibitors of acid secretion. In severe GORD, relapse is extremely common, and usually occurs within days of stopping treatment.

2. A benign oesophageal stricture has developed, with the acute presentation of food bolus obstruction. Stricture formation is one of the complications of GORD (others being oesophageal ulceration and Barrett's oesophagus) and may be associated with the relief of reflux symptoms.

3. Carcinoma of the oesophagus, oesophageal dysmotility (such as a nutcracker oesophagus), achalasia of the oesophagus and oesophageal webs. In oesophageal carcinoma the dysphagia presents gradually over a period of a few months, may be more pronounced for solids than liquids, and is usually associated with significant weight loss.

   Oesophageal dysmotility syndromes are not necessarily associated with reflux symptoms; there should be no weight loss but there may be odynophagia (pain on swallowing).

   It may be difficult to differentiate achalasia from either oesophageal carcinoma or benign oesophageal stricture. Typically, the dysphagia in achalasia is for both solids and liquids, but dysphagia for solids may predominate. It may be associated with marked weight loss and can occur at any age, although it is rare in children.

   Distal oesophageal webs may be associated with a typical history of 'restaurant dysphagia', characterized by acute dysphagia, vomiting, and then the ability to continue the remainder of the meal without any further difficulty.

CASE 2

Emilia Pintez is a 32-year-old Puerto Rican, resident in the USA for the past 5 years and currently employed as a live-in nanny for two boisterous children. Her employer, a leading figure in local social awareness issues, notices that Emilia has been coughing up frank blood for the past two weeks and, concerned about tuberculosis, insists on her attending the local clinic. Emilia reports that she is not overly concerned: she has coughed up blood intermittently "for the past two months". However, she has noticed that it has become increasingly difficult to keep up with the children and get to her attic room without pausing for a break. She also reports waking up in the middle of night "short of breath and coughing". Other than a poorly remembered childhood illness (she vaguely recalls that she couldn't walk properly), no other medical history was elicited.

QUESTIONS

1. If you were the family doctor, would you advise screening of the children for tuberculosis? If not, why not?

2. How would you grade Emilia's exercise tolerance?

3. What symptom is Emilia describing when she complains of shortness of breath?

4. What is a possible diagnosis from the history?

NOTES FOR REVISION

YOUR ANSWERS

1 Would screening of the children for tuberculosis be advisable, and, if not, why not?

2 Grading of Emilia's exercise tolerance

3 Emilia's symptom when she complains of shortness of breath

4 Possible diagnosis from the history

ANSWERS

6.12, 6.13, 6.14, 7.20, 7.39

1. No. It is inappropriate to jump to conclusions prior to examination of the patient. Haemoptysis may be due to a number of conditions, including cardiac, respiratory and haematological causes. Although tuberculosis should never be overlooked as a cause of haemoptysis, the patient's history strongly suggests that a cardiac cause for the haemoptysis will be found on examination.

2. New York Heart Association Grade 2. An aide-mémoire to this very useful functional assessment of the severity of cardiac failure is the key word 'ordinary'. The patient's dyspnoea may then be graded according to whether they are dyspnoeic with more than ordinary activity (Grade 1), with ordinary activity (Grade 2), less than ordinary activity (Grade 3) or at rest (Grade 4).

3. Paroxysmal nocturnal dyspnoea (PND). PND is cardiac in origin, and represents an exacerbation of left ventricular failure brought about by adoption of the supine position and sleep. There are two postulated mechanisms. First, the mobilization of oedema when supine and a relative drop in urine production leads to an increase in intravascular volume sufficient to further compromise a failing heart. Second, an increased sympathetic drive (perhaps while dreaming) shortens the time for diastolic filling, leading to a further increase in end diastolic atrial pressures.

4. Mitral stenosis secondary to rheumatic heart disease. Rheumatic heart disease must be excluded in any young patient who presents with symptoms of dyspnoea upon exertion, PND and haemoptysis (which in the setting of mitral stenosis may be due to bronchial vein rupture, bronchitis or left ventricular failure), and even more so in a patient brought up in a Third World country where socio-economic conditions predispose to rheumatic fever.

CASE 3

Stella Jones, a 19-year-old student, attends the university clinic, worried that she might be jaundiced and complaining that she "just doesn't feel right". She is concerned that the two problems might be linked to her drinking far more alcohol than usual during the student induction week, but she cannot quantify exactly how much she drank. She feels that her non-specific ill health has been exacerbated by the poor quality of food in the student canteen. The proof of this, she claims, is the deterioration of her skin back to the "pimple factory" days of her youth. Finally, she is concerned that she might be pregnant: she has missed her periods for the past 4 months.

QUESTIONS

1. What further details relating to her jaundice would you like to know?

2. What would you look for on examination?

3. Apart from pregnancy, what other causes of secondary amenorrhoea should be considered?

4. What diagnosis should be considered?

NOTES FOR REVISION

YOUR ANSWERS

1 Further details relating to Stella's jaundice

2 What to look for on examination

3 Causes of secondary amenorrhoea, other than pregnancy, to be considered

4 Diagnosis to be considered

ANSWERS

1. In the patient with jaundice, a number of direct questions must be asked to determine both the underlying cause and the chronicity of the problem. Thus enquiries are made about alcohol abuse, blood transfusions or intravenous drug abuse (hepatitis C); homosexuality (hepatitis B); medications, contact with jaundiced patients or travel to areas with endemic hepatitis A; itching (cholestatic liver disease); weight loss and pain (malignancy).

2. The examination of a patient who is jaundiced should be aimed towards answering three questions. First, is the liver disease acute or chronic? Look for the cutaneous stigmata of chronic liver disease (clubbed fingers, white nails, palmar erythema, Dupuytren's contracture, gynaecomastia, spider naevi). Second, is there evidence of decompensated liver disease (jaundice, ascites, encephalopathy)? Third, are there any clues as to the underlying aetiology such as tattoos (hepatitis B), slate coloured skin (haemochromatosis), azure blue lunulae or Kayser–Fleischer rings (Wilson's disease)?

3. The periodicity of the menstrual cycle is notoriously unreliable, and vulnerable to the effects of stress, anxiety, fear of pregnancy, as well as a wide range of organic disorders. In a patient who has non-specific ill health and jaundice, constitutional diseases must be considered, in particular chronic illnesses and autoimmune diseases.

4. Autoimmune hepatitis (synonym: chronic active hepatitis). The possibility that a jaundiced patient has underlying chronic liver disease should always be considered and excluded, and especially so in a young jaundiced girl who also has the features of non-specific ill health, acne and amenorrhoea.

CASE 4

Derwin Trotter, a 47-year-old journalist, consults his doctor complaining despairingly that life has become intolerable since the recurrence of the most severe headaches he has ever known. He describes being woken in the night by an excruciatingly sharp pain in the left eyeball, akin to the "slow insertion of an icepick". The eye is reddened and waters intensely. His nose feels blocked. The duration of the acute pain is variable, lasting from minutes to half an hour. After each episode (he has had seven in the past 2 weeks) he feels exhausted, but suffers no residual headache. He reports experiencing identical headaches 5 years before, but these lasted for 5 days only and then disappeared. He is otherwise well. He smokes 20 cigarettes per day. The doctor finds no abnormalities on examination, is uncertain about the diagnosis, but thinks the patient may be suffering from migraine. However, he is called to the patient's house early one morning, observes the patient during an acute attack and notes that the left eye is watering excessively and that his pupils are unequal.

QUESTIONS

1. What are the causes of unequal pupils?

2. What is the cause of this patient's unequal pupils, and what are the other causes of this syndrome?

3. Headaches are usually diagnosed from the history, and examination is usually non-contributory. What is the diagnosis in this patient?

NOTES FOR REVISION

YOUR ANSWERS

1 Causes of unequal pupils

2 Cause of Mr Trotter's unequal pupils and other causes of this syndrome

3 Diagnosis in Mr Trotter from the history

ANSWERS

1. Unequal pupils may be normal, and patients should be asked if they have noticed them before (they usually have). Pathologically unequal pupils may be due to (i) diseases affecting the sympathetic innervation of the pupil, thus giving a unilateral miotic pupil (Horner's syndrome), (ii) diseases affecting the parasympathetic innervation of the pupil via the third nerve, thus giving a unilateral dilated pupil (posterior communicating artery aneurysm, midbrain vascular lesion, any cause of mononeuritis multiplex, midbrain demyelinating lesion), (iii) disease affecting the midbrain giving unequal small and irregular pupils (Argyll Robertson pupil) and finally (iv) the tonic pupil syndrome, of unclear aetiology, where the affected pupil is dilated but becomes progressively smaller with time.

2. The patient has Horner's syndrome (miosis, ptosis, enophthalmos). This results from interruption of the sympathetic innervation to the eye. The ocular sympathetic supply runs a lengthy course from the hypothalamus down the spinal cord, exiting at nerve roots C8–T2, coursing across the apex of the lung, under the subclavian artery and then travelling with the internal carotid to the ophthalmic artery and thence to the iris, via the nasociliary nerve. A lesion anywhere along this route can give rise to Horner's syndrome, for example cervical lesions, apical lung neoplasm, and inflammatory vasculitis.

3. Cluster headaches. The presenting history is so typical of cluster headaches, and indeed the cluster headache symptom complex is so specific, that usually no further investigation is justified. The physical signs during an attack are limited to the affected eye becoming red and watery, the ipsilateral nostril either feeling blocked or running, and an ipsilateral Horner's syndrome in 30% of cases. Most sufferers have bouts (clusters) of headaches occurring over a period of days or weeks, with complete absence for months or even years. Such a pattern is called episodic cluster headache. In 20% of patients, however, the attacks occur regularly without break (chronic cluster headache).

   There are no diagnostic tests for cluster headaches.

CASE 5

A home visit is requested by Steven Galevich, a 56-year-old author. He describes an unusual sequence of events. Whilst absorbed by the intricacies of a murder scene in his latest novel, he flung his head into his hands for further contemplation, and was distracted by a loud crack from his right arm. He complains of ongoing pain, which is eased by analgesics. What also bothers him, however, is a continual thirst and endless trips to the lavatory to pass urine, all of which interrupts his creative process. In addition, despite these visits to the lavatory he has not had a bowel motion for the past 6 days, and feels uncomfortable about his stomach. His wife adds that he is particularly irritable, though not much more than normal!

QUESTIONS

1. What electrolyte abnormality should be considered?

2. What is the cause of this patient's bone pain?

3. What is the most likely diagnosis, and what has caused the metabolic abnormality?

NOTES FOR REVISION

YOUR ANSWERS

1 Electrolyte abnormality to be considered

2 Cause of Mr Galevich's bone pain

3 Most likely diagnosis in Mr Galavich, and what has caused the metabolic abnormality

ANSWERS

3.16, 11.9

1. Hypercalcaemia. He supplies a history of thirst, polyuria, constipation and abdominal pain. Although individually non-specific, in combination these symptoms are suggestive of hypercalcaemia (other symptoms include anorexia, nausea, vomiting, proximal muscle weakness, depression and confusion).

2. A pathological fracture of the humerus. Bone pain may be either diffuse (due to multiple bone secondaries, Paget's disease of the bone, osteoporosis or osteomalacia) or focal (due to fracture, trauma, osteomyelitis, focal metastatic deposits and osteogenic tumours). In this patient he sustained a fracture with minimal trauma, which is highly suggestive of a pathological fracture. Pathological fractures may occur in the setting of focal metastatic deposits (in particular breast and prostatic cancer) or diffuse malignant bone involvement (multiple myeloma).

3. Multiple myeloma. Although there are a number of causes of hypercalcaemia (hyperparathyroidism, malignancy associated, medication induced or secondary to granulomatous diseases and endocrinopathies) the combination of a pathological fracture and hypercalcaemia in a male makes myeloma the most likely.

   The hypercalcaemia in multiple myeloma is due to production of osteoclast-activating factor by the malignant plasma cell clone.

CASE 6

Paula Apple, a 56-year-old woman, had primary biliary cirrhosis diagnosed 12 years ago. Owing to a significant rise in her bilirubin level, a further deterioration in the synthetic function of her liver and generalized tiredness she was considered for a liver transplant. On examining the patient prior to transplant, a final-year medical student noted that she had clubbed fingers, white nails, xanthelasma and numerous spider naevi. The liver transplant was performed successfully a few weeks later but grave complications ensued, requiring two admissions to the intensive therapy unit, and one laparotomy for surgical revision of a biliary stricture. Five months after the procedure she is making a slow recovery. She is seen by the former student, now an intern on the unit, who notes that her fingers are no longer clubbed, that the white nails have disappeared, but that she now has two transverse ridges across her nails.

QUESTIONS

1. Why do patients with cirrhosis get white nails, and is this clinical sign distinct from leuconychia?

2. What other nail changes may be seen in cirrhosis?

3. What is the eponym attached to the transverse ridges in the nails, and what is the aetiology?

1 Why patients with cirrhosis get white nails, and whether this sign is distinct from leuconychia

2 Other nail changes that may be seen in cirrhosis

3 Eponym attached to the transverse ridges in the nails and its aetiology

NOTES FOR REVISION

ANSWERS

4.24, 4.26, 4.3

1. In the normal nail a translucent nail plate lies on top of a highly vascular nail bed, thus giving the nail its pink appearance. In cirrhosis, in the presence of hypoalbuminaemia, the nail bed becomes opacified thus giving a white nail appearance. In contrast leuconychia is due to whiteness of the nail plate. Leuconychia may be either congenital (autosomal dominant, may be associated with deafness) or acquired. Acquired leuconychia may be associated with general medical diseases and may be acute, as in the white stripes seen in arsenic poisoning (Mees' lines).

2. Hypoalbuminaemia may give rise to Muehrcke's lines (paired narrow white bands lying transversely across the nail). Again, these are not due to changes in the nail plate.

3. Beau's lines. These are transverse ridges or depressions in the nail plate which occur when there are interruptions in the growth of the nail (during severe illness, for example).

CASE 7

Sandy Alday, a 28-year-old doctor, arranges to see a dermatologist. She complains that over the past 3 weeks she has developed an itchy rash over her body. The itching is worse over her buttocks, breasts and armpits and particularly severe after a hot bath. As she was doing a haematology rotation at the time, she had checked her full blood count, which was normal. Despite a change in her washing powder and extensive use of lanolin cream the itching persisted, driving her – and her husband! – to distraction. She is on no medications, and has no past medical history apart from childhood hay fever. She has not travelled recently, except to a nearby resort 5 weeks ago for a temporary hospital attachment. On examination she is well presented and well nourished. She is not jaundiced. There is an eczematous rash over her buttocks, breasts, axillae and periumbilical region, with marked excoriation over the buttocks and areas of secondary infection and pustulation. The head, face, palms and soles are spared. Infected eczema is suspected, and she is given an unsuccessful trial of topical corticosteroids and systemic antibiotics. A number of other specialists are called in, all of whom are convinced that the problem is primarily dermatological. A skin biopsy is finally performed, revealing the diagnosis.

QUESTIONS

1. What systemic, non-dermatological diseases cause pruritus?

2. What types of eczematous dermatitis have been described?

3. What diagnosis was revealed by the skin biopsy?

YOUR ANSWERS

1 Systemic, non-dermatological diseases causing pruritus

2 Types of eczematous dermatitis described

3 Diagnosis revealed by skin biopsy

NOTES FOR REVISION

ANSWERS

4.4, 4.11–4.16, 4.20

1. Generalized pruritus without diagnostic skin lesions may occur in endocrine diseases (diabetes, hyperthyroidism, carcinoid), malignancy (lymphoma), haematological diseases (leukaemia, polycythaemia and mastocytosis), chronic renal failure, cholestasis and may occasionally be psychogenic in origin.

2. Eczematous dermatitis is not a specific disease entity, and describes merely a characteristic inflammatory response of the skin to both exogenous and endogenous agents. The distribution of the skin lesions and the suspected pathogenesis allows for the recognition of a variety of types of eczematous dermatitis, such as atopic, allergic contact, asteatotic and nummular eczematous dermatitis, stasis and seborrhoeic dermatitis and lichen simplex chronicus.

3. Scabies, acquired from unwashed linen during her temporary hospital post. Type IV sensitization to the 'itch mite', *Sarcoptes scabiei*, occurs approximately 1 month after infection. This can lead to either a papular or eczematous reaction at the site of infestation.

CASE 8

Samuel Richman, a 60-year-old publisher, makes an appointment to see his doctor. He reports that over the past 6 or 7 months he has noticed a general decline in fitness, such that he is no longer able to do the weekly food shopping unassisted. Associated with this is an annoying cough (which does not "bring anything up"). He had stopped smoking at age 59. He reports no history suggestive of any neurological problem or Raynaud's phenomenon, has no other medical or surgical history and takes no medications. He is not a pet owner and has not travelled recently. On examination he is apyrexial and his fingers clearly clubbed. The doctor thinks he is cyanosed. No skin rashes or infiltrations are visible. He has no pedal oedema, his jugular venous pressure (JVP) is not elevated and there is no cardiomegaly, or additional heart sounds or murmurs. On chest examination, he had marked bilateral basal mid and late inspiratory crackles.

QUESTIONS

1. What is the significance of the past and social history?

2. How would you define cyanosis, and what is the differential diagnosis?

3. How accurate is the clinical appreciation of central cyanosis?

4. What simple examination techniques can be used to help confirm the clinical impression of clubbing?

5. What is the most likely diagnosis in this patient?

NOTES FOR REVISION

YOUR ANSWERS

1 Significance of the past and social history

2 Definition of cyanosis and its differential diagnosis

3 Accuracy of the clinical appreciation of central cyanosis

4 Simple examination techniques to help confirm the clinical impression of clubbing

5 Most likely diagnosis in Mr Richman

ANSWERS

1. The history will help exclude autoimmune, drug-associated and extrinsic allergic disorders, alveolitis and asbestosis.

2. Cyanosis by definition refers to a bluish discoloration of the skin and mucous membranes. This discoloration may be due either to the presence of reduced (unsaturated) haemoglobin in the capillary blood (> 5 g/dl in capillary blood) or to the presence of increased amounts of haemoglobin derivatives in the capillary blood. The differential diagnosis of cyanosis must therefore include the causes of decreased arterial oxygen saturation (decreased atmospheric pressure, impaired pulmonary function, anatomic shunts and haemoglobin variants with a low affinity for oxygen) as well as the haemoglobin abnormalities which give a bluish discoloration of the skin indistinguishable from that due to impaired oxygen saturation (methaemoglobinaemia, sulfhaemoglobinaemia).

3. The clinical assessment of cyanosis is poor. Greater than 5 g/dl of reduced haemoglobin corresponds to a saturation of 85%. In a study of cyanosis as a physical sign, 25% of experienced observers recorded definitely no cyanosis in 20 patients with oxygen saturation below 75%, and 32% recorded definite cyanosis in 20 patients who had saturations greater than 96%.

4. When normal nails are placed 'back to back' a diamond-shaped area is created. In clubbing this is obliterated.

5. The combination of clubbing, cyanosis and end inspiratory crackles is very suggestive of interstitial lung disease. To make the diagnosis of cryptogenic fibrosing alveolitis, the known causes of interstitial lung disease (environmental toxins, drugs, radiation, poisons) must be excluded. You should also look for evidence of collagen-vascular disease (in clubbing rheumatoid disease) which may be associated with similar chest findings.

CASE 9

Jonas Kowalski, a 68-year-old mechanic, is referred to a specialist unit by his doctor. He first presented 4 months ago, complaining of an itchy, scaly rash on his back. Contact dermatitis was diagnosed and the patient reassured. The rash on his back disappeared, but a few days later discrete scaly lesions appeared over his trunk, arms and thighs. He consults his doctor again who thinks this time that the lesions are compatible with a particular presentation of psoriasis. However, the patient does not give a history of recent sore throat and also mentions that the lesions are itchy. Nonetheless, no specific treatment is recommended and indeed the rash resolves over a few weeks.

QUESTIONS

1. What diseases should be considered in patients presenting with scaly skin lesions?

2. What presentation of psoriasis is the family doctor diagnosing?

3. What alternative diagnosis should be considered?

NOTES FOR REVISION

YOUR ANSWERS

1 Diseases to be considered in patients presenting with scaly skin lesions

2 Presentation of psoriasis diagnosed by the family doctor

3 Alternative diagnosis to be considered

ANSWERS

4.9, 4.14–4.15

1. Scaling macules or papules may be seen in drug-induced hypersensitivity reactions, psoriasis, secondary syphilis, pityriasis rosea, dermatophytosis (ringworm infections) and candidiasis. Psoriasiform lesions may also be seen in Reiter's syndrome (keratoderma blennorrhagicum), cutaneous T-cell lymphoma, and nummular eczema.

2. Guttate psoriasis. In this presentation, which may follow acute streptococcal pharyngitis, the lesions are 1–3 cm in size, well defined, slightly raised and erythematous. Guttate psoriasis may either resolve or persist as chronic psoriasis.

3. Pityriasis rosea. The initial single lesion on the patient's back was the 'herald patch', which appears a few days before the generalized rash. The generalized rash consists of itchy, 1–3 cm macules with a 'shirt and shorts' distribution, and fades spontaneously over 6 weeks.

CASE 10

Myra Levinsky, a 47-year-old New Yorker, visits her son in London. Four days after arrival she is admitted to the local emergency department. She feels tired and weak, feverish, and complains of mouth ulcers. She has no past medical history of note. Prior to departure, she had discovered a bottle of sleeping tablets used by her aged mother and taken two tablets to help her sleep throughout the flight. On examination, she looks ill and is pyrexial. She has vivid, erythematous skin lesions on her legs and hands, together with occasional bullae. There are blisters on her buccal mucosae, and ulcers on her gingivae. The rest of her examination is non-contributory.

QUESTIONS

1. What diseases are associated with the development of skin vesicles and/or bullae?

2. What two important bullous diseases should be considered in this patient, and what are the putative causes?

3. What characteristic skin signs are described in these two conditions?

NOTES FOR REVISION

YOUR ANSWERS

1 Diseases associated with skin vesicles and/or bullae

2 Two important bullous diseases to be considered in Myra and their putative causes

3 Characteristic skin signs described in these two conditions

ANSWERS

4.10, 4.21

1. Vesicle and/or bullae formation are the major feature of a number of infections, both viral (rickettsial pox, varicella, herpes zoster, disseminated herpes simplex, enterovirus) and bacterial (staphylococcal scalded skin syndrome); allergic contact dermatitis (such as with poison ivy); thermal injury; and the bullous diseases of unknown cause (pemphigus and pemphigoid).

   Vesicles and/or bullae are also associated with, but not necessarily, the predominant feature of, erythema multiforme and porphyria cutanea tarda.

2. Erythema multiforme and pemphigus. In erythema multiforme no cause is found in 50% of cases. Possible aetiological agents in the remaining cases include herpes virus, *Mycoplasma pneumoniae* and drugs (penicillins, barbiturates, phenytoin, sulphonamides). In the above case, erythema multiforme should be considered given the history of 'a sleeping tablet', later ascertained to be a barbiturate.

   Pemphigus is an autoimmune disorder of unknown aetiology, characterized by an IgG response to an intercellular constituent of the epidermal cells, leading to intraepithelial acantholysis.

3. The target lesion is typical of erythema multiforme, but is not always seen. In pemphigus, Nikolsky's sign can be elicited.

3

CASE 11

Danny Baker, a 61-year-old glazier and ardent football fan, reports that at the previous two games, both within the last 3 weeks, he has been unable to join in the cheering with his usual fervour. He has not noticed any other change to his voice. As for past history, he reports that he used to suffer from heartburn, but this has completely resolved since starting a new antacid capsule. He also recalls a sexually acquired disease, diagnosed and treated 40 years ago during a 2-year stay in Australia. He smokes 25–30 cigarettes per day. His weight is stable. On examination he has a brownish-black discoloration of the posterior surface of the tongue. No other buccal, oral or throat lesions are noted. Nothing else of note is found on general examination.

QUESTIONS

1. What is the probable cause of Mr Baker's tongue discoloration. In general, what other morphological and colour changes affecting the tongue are described?

2. What differential diagnosis for his voice problem would you consider?

YOUR ANSWERS

1 Probable cause of Mr Baker's tongue discoloration

2 Differential diagnosis for Mr Baker's voice problem

CASE 12

Richard Caines, a 38-year-old cardiologist, is particularly proud of his auscultatory prowess, and disdainful of those who insist on 'waiting for the echocardiogram'. He is therefore dismayed at missing a mid-diastolic murmur, which is picked up instead by the intern. A few minutes earlier he was aware of a fullness in the left ear, as if he had just come out of the shower. On starting to discuss the management plan with the team, he is suddenly overcome with vertigo, and forced to sit down. This takes the patient and his colleagues by surprise, especially as he looks close to vomiting. After a few minutes the cardiologist stands up and continues the ward visit. A few hours later, sitting at his desk, he again feels a fullness in his ear, followed by profound vertigo, which this time lasts 30 minutes. He sees a colleague in the ear, nose and throat department, and on crude testing is found to be slightly deaf in the left ear. Weber's test is performed, and the patient can hear the vibration better in the right ear. On formal neurological testing no abnormality is found.

QUESTIONS

1. From Weber's test, did the patient have a conductive or sensorineural deafness?

2. In this type of deafness, would the Rinne test be positive or negative?

3. What is the most likely diagnosis?

YOUR ANSWERS

1 Does the Weber test indicate a conductive or sensorineural deafness?

2 In this type of deafness, would the Rinne test be positive?

3 Most likely diagnosis in Richard?

ANSWERS TO CASE 11

3.25, 5.7

1. A black tongue may be due to drugs, such as liquid bismuth preparations, smoking, and the sucking or eating of a suitably dark chromogenic substance. Other colour changes described in the tongue are (i) the geographic tongue (appearance of denuded red patches wandering across the tongue due to loss and regrowth of filiform papillae), (ii) the strawberry tongue seen in scarlet fever (due to hypertrophy of the fungiform papillae), (iii) the bald tongue seen in pernicious anaemia, pellagra and syphilis (due to atrophy of the papillae). Morphological changes seen are macroglossia (found in Down's syndrome, acromegaly, amyloid and local tumor), and the fissured 'scrotal' tongue.

2. Squamous carcinoma of the larynx is the most common tumour of the larynx, and should be excluded in any patient with hoarseness of over two weeks' duration, especially in smokers. From his history other possibilities would include simple overuse of the voice, chronic vocal abuse with the formation of nodules on the vocal cords, and tertiary syphilis. Chronic reflux of gastric acid may cause hoarseness, coughing (worse at night) and asthma.

ANSWERS TO CASE 12

5.2, 12.56

1. A sensorineural deafness. With Weber's test in a unilateral conductive defect, the vibration is perceived better in the affected ear. In a sensorineural loss vibration is perceived better in the unaffected ear.

2. The Rinne test is reported as positive if air conduction is found to be better than bone conduction, and negative when the reverse occurs. In sensorineural loss both air and bone conduction perception are reduced, but air conduction is still heard louder – as it is in normal hearing. Thus the Rinne test would be reported as positive.

3. Menière's disease. The combination of a fullness/plugged sensation in the affected ear together with relapsing and remitting episodes of hearing impairment and vertigo is a typical presentation. The prognosis is variable, and although the dizzy spells disappear within 12–18 months, some hearing impairment can remain, and in 20% of patients the condition eventually becomes bilateral.

CASE 13

Arnie Pompost, an unmarried 46-year-old architect and wine taster, enjoys showing off his expertise at social gatherings. A week ago, at a long-awaited gathering of equal-minded *bons vivants* (ostensibly to celebrate the latest Museum of Modern Art exhibition) he notes with some horror that he has a blocked nose, and cannot smell. He has no other symptoms, but seeks an urgent appointment with a specialist. His mind is put at rest with a simple diagnosis. Over the next few days, however, Mr Pompost becomes progressively more blocked up, with a runny nose. He revisits his specialist, complaining of pain below his right eye. He has a feeling of intense pressure in that region, almost as if it were about to explode, worse on bending forward. On examination he is found to be apyrexial, and exquisitely tender to pressure over the right cheekbone anteriorly. He has purulent mucus from both nostrils. Nothing else of note is found.

QUESTIONS

1. What is your approach to the patient who cannot smell?

2. What is the most likely cause of this patient's anosmia?

3. What complication has developed?

4. What unusual complications may further develop?

NOTES FOR REVISION

YOUR ANSWERS

1 Approach to the patient who cannot smell

2 Most likely cause of Mr Pompost's anosmia

3 Complication that has developed

4 Unusual complications that may further develop

ANSWERS

5.3, 5.9–5.10, 12.15

1. A problem with smelling (hyposmia, total or partial anosmia) may be due to (i) processes preventing access of the odourant to the olfactory neuroepithelium (acute viral or bacterial rhinitis, allergic rhinitis, deviated nasal septum), (ii) sensory loss due to damage of the sensory epithelium (postviral infections, neoplasms, toxins, cranial irradiation), and (iii) disruption of the central olfactory pathways (head trauma, neoplasms of the anterior cribriform plate, marble bone disease and congenital disorders such as Kallmann's syndrome).

2. An acute upper respiratory viral infection, with rhinitis, is the most likely cause. Usually transient, the sensory epithelium may rarely be destroyed and replaced with scar tissue leading to permanent postviral anosmia.

3. A bacterial superinfection, with development of acute maxillary sinusitis.

4. Complications of frontal sinusitis include osteomyelitis of the skull base, meningitis, epidural abscess, brain abscess and cavernous sinus thrombosis.

CASE 14

The medical intern is called to see a patient in the resuscitation bay. Paul Hedges, a 56-year-old man, has well-documented chronic obstructive airways disease, and still smokes 20 cigarettes per day. He is quite lucid when seen, but clearly very short of breath. He says that at best he can walk 50 yards on the flat before needing to rest, but that for the most part he is housebound. For the past week he has been coughing up yellow-green sputum, a change from the usual off-white phlegm which he has coughed up for most of the year (and indeed for a number of years previously). For the past 2 days he has been short of breath at rest. The intern notes that the patient is cyanosed despite being placed on oxygen by the nurses. During examination the patient becomes less and less coherent, and eventually unrousable. Assistance is sought.

QUESTIONS

1. What two facts may be inferred from the history of productive cough?

2. What should the doctor look for in this patient on examination?

3. What caused the patient to become less coherent and lose consciousness?

<table>
<tr><td>YOUR ANSWERS</td></tr>
<tr><td>1 The two facts that may be inferred from the history of productive cough</td></tr>
<tr><td>2 What the doctor should look for on examination of Mr Hedges</td></tr>
<tr><td>3 What caused Mr Hedges to become less coherent and lose consciousness</td></tr>
</table>

CASE 15

Albertina Serthole, a 46-year-old lady, complains that over the past few weeks her general energy and fitness have slowly deteriorated, such that at present she finds she is breathless on minimal exertion. She does not report a cough or chest pain, and indeed has no past respiratory or cardiovascular problems. She has never smoked, and takes no medications other than tamoxifen. This was begun 3 years ago after undergoing a lumpectomy for a growth in her left breast.

QUESTIONS

1. What questions need answering by the examination?

2. What are the signs of a pleural effusion?

<table>
<tr><td>YOUR ANSWERS</td></tr>
<tr><td>1 Questions that need answering by the examination</td></tr>
<tr><td>2 Signs of pleural effusion</td></tr>
</table>

6.8–6.9, 6.13, 6.21, 6.25

ANSWERS TO CASE 14

1. First, that he has chronic obstructive bronchitis, and second that he has acquired a lower respiratory infection. Epidemiologically, chronic bronchitis is defined as the production of sputum for 3 consecutive months in 2 successive years. The history is compatible with this. The change in colour of sputum suggests either acute bronchitis or pneumonia. The yellow sputum may be due to the presence of leucocytes, changing to green from the action of an enzyme, verdoperoxidase. These colour changes may be due to eosinophils, and not indicate infection, but this finding is usually restricted to acute asthma rather than the chronic bronchitic.

2. The evidence indicates that the patient belongs to the blue bloater spectrum of chronic obstructive airways disease (he has chronic bronchitis, is cyanosed, has cor pulmonale and deteriorates on oxygen therapy). These patients are usually overweight, polycythaemic with or without cyanosis, have features of carbon dioxide retention (dilated superficial veins, asterixis, papilloedema), are not particularly short of breath at rest (especially in comparison to the pink puffers) and have cor pulmonale. The clinical features of cor pulmonale include evidence of right heart overload (a left parasternal heave, tricuspid regurgitation), pulmonary hypertension (a palpable P2), a raised JVP with or without V waves, a palpable, tender liver which may or may not be pulsatile, and lower limb oedema. This fluid retention is secondary to hypoxia-induced renal salt and water retention, and responds to correction of the hypoxia.

3. The oxygen therapy. Blue bloaters respond to hypoxia by increasing their red blood cell mass to increase oxygen delivery, and resetting their medullary chemoreceptors to have a normal ventilatory response to a higher $PaCO_2$. They are then dependent on hypoxic ventilatory drive from the less sensitive peripheral carotid receptors. The injudicious use of high inspired oxygen concentration can switch off this ventilatory stimulus.

ANSWERS TO CASE 15

6.32, 6.33

1. It is necessary to establish whether her symptoms are likely to be due to recurrence/dissemination of the tumour or some other lung disease. You should therefore look for evidence of local recurrence of the carcinoma or enlargement of lymph nodes. In the lungs, dissemination of tumour will either be as multiple intrapulmonary deposits (which will not be detectable clinically) or a pleural effusion. Other common conditions to be excluded are airways disease and lung fibrosis. Consider also anaemia, heart failure and pulmonary emboli.

2. The reporting of the findings on examination of the respiratory system should follow the inspection, palpation, percussion and auscultation approach. On inspection, excursion of the affected side may be limited due to underlying compression of the lung. On palpation, vocal fremitus will be decreased. On percussion, stony dullness over the affected area will be detected. Finally, on auscultation breath sounds will be reduced and there may be bronchial breathing at the top of the effusion. If you have difficulty in distinguishing the dullness of consolidation from the stony dullness of fluid remember that in consolidation vocal fremitus will be increased and bronchial breathing will be heard.

CASE 16

Michael Stalinki, an 18-year-old engineering student with a history of asthma, is playing an interfaculty football match when he becomes aware that his chest is tighter than usual, and breathing more difficult. Despite medication, his wheeze becomes more pronounced and he goes to the nearby hospital. He is assessed, treated and discharged within 4 hours. He remains well for the next 4 months. During a lecture he suddenly becomes aware of a stabbing pain in the left side of his chest. He also feels nauseated and short of breath. The pain abates somewhat but his breathing deteriorates rapidly, despite use of his asthma medication. By the time he arrives in the emergency room he has great difficulty in breathing. A quick examination reveals that he is cyanosed, his trachea deviated to the right, and breath sounds are minimal over the left lung field. A life-saving procedure is performed.

QUESTIONS

1. What clinical findings should have been documented when the patient first attended hospital?

2. What caused his sudden deterioration 4 months later, and what life-saving procedure was done?

3. What are the other known causes of this problem?

4. What other conditions result in tracheal deviation?

NOTES FOR REVISION

YOUR ANSWERS

1 Clinical findings that should have been documented when Michael first attended hospital

2 What caused Michael's sudden deterioration 4 months later, and what life-saving procedure was done

3 Other known causes of this problem

4 Other conditions that result in tracheal deviation

ANSWERS

6.6, 6.19, 6.20, 6.21, 6.24, 6.25–6.26, 6.30, 6.32

1. The signs and symptoms that indicate a severe asthma attack are an inability to complete sentences, a respiratory rate greater than 25 breaths/min, a pulse rate greater than 110 beats/min, pulsus paradoxus, peak expiratory flow rate, cyanosis and a silent chest on auscultation.

2. A tension pneumothorax. A pneumothorax alone would not result in tracheal deviation or, in a healthy individual, cyanosis. A large bore needle was inserted into the chest, prior to insertion of a chest drain.

3. The causes of pneumothorax may be either spontaneous or traumatic. The latter may be iatrogenic (ventilation, central line insertion, post-thoracentesis, post-transbronchial biopsy etc.), or may occur from penetrating or non-penetrating chest trauma. Spontaneous pneumothoraces may occur in the setting of asthma, chronic obstruction airways disease, malignancy, interstitial lung disease and cystic fibrosis, or be idiopathic.

4. The trachea may be either pushed or pulled away from the normal midline position. It is pushed away from the side of a tension pneumothorax, or by very large pleural effusion. It is pulled towards the side of apical collapse or fibrosis.

CASE 17

Tony Crabtree, a 63-year-old man, is sent as an urgent referral to the admitting medical team. He complains of having a headache for the past 3 weeks. The headache is diffuse, unremitting, and no longer responds to analgesics. He has not noticed any weakness, loss of balance or clumsiness, does not complain of a stiff neck, and has not suffered any head trauma. He feels 'full' in the face, and his wife remarks that his face looks more puffy and red than normal. On examination there are distended superficial veins, the jugular venous pressure is elevated, his face is plethoric with periorbital puffiness, and there is chemosis. The trachea is central, but lymphadenopathy is palpated in the supraclavicular region. The fingers are not clubbed. On examination of the chest a wheeze is heard, possibly localized over the right anterior chest wall. The rest of the examination is normal.

QUESTIONS

1. What syndrome is this patient presenting with, and what are the two most common causes?

2. Why does the patient not have clubbed fingers?

3. Describe five clinical problems that could result from regional spread of the most common cause of this patient's syndrome.

NOTES FOR REVISION

YOUR ANSWERS

1 Mr Crabtree's syndrome and its two most common causes

2 Why the patient does not have clubbed fingers

3 Five clinical problems resulting from regional spread of the most common cause of Mr Crabtree's syndrome

ANSWERS

1. Superior vena cava syndrome. This results from obstruction of the superior vena cava due to compression or infiltration by tumours in the superior mediastinum. The above presentation is a typical one. In the vast majority the underlying cause is a malignant process, and in about 75% of cases the malignancy is lung cancer. In nearly all of the remaining 25% the malignancy is a lymphoma. Very rarely the syndrome may be due to fibrosing mediastinitis (idiopathic, or secondary to methysergide and histoplasmosis).

2. The most common lung cancers are squamous cell (a third), adenocarcinoma (a quarter) and small cell (a quarter). Clubbing of fingers is not always present and is rare in small cell neoplasms. This is probably because the rate of growth in small cell cancer is so rapid that the patient will have requested medical attention prior to the development of clubbed fingers. Hypertrophic pulmonary osteoarthropathy (i.e. clubbing with periostitis) is usually seen with adenocarcinoma.

3. Regional spread of lung cancer leads to a number of well-described presentations. These include (i) dysphagia (oesophageal compression), (ii) hoarseness (recurrent laryngeal nerve compression), (ii) dyspnoea (phrenic nerve paralysis and elevation of the hemidiaphragm, lymphatic obstruction with a pleural effusion, lymphangitis carcinomatosa), (iii) Horner's syndrome (sympathetic nerve paralysis), (iv) shoulder and arm pain in the distribution of the ulnar nerve in Pancoast's syndrome (involvement of C8, T1, T2 roots and destruction of first and second ribs), and (v) cardiac tamponade (pericardial invasion), arrhythmias and cardiac failure (cardiac involvement).

CASE 18

Amos is a 34-year-old biochemist, basket-ball player and amateur trumpeter. He collapsed with chest pain whilst playing the trumpet at a friend's stag night party, and has been brought to casualty. On examination he looks worried, restless and in pain. He can't find a comfortable position to lie in. He describes a sudden tearing pain which started between his shoulderblades, and he now has discomfort in his chest, his jaw and his right arm. He is a keep-fit fanatic and doesn't smoke. His knowledge of family history is sketchy as many relatives died in the war. On examination he is pale and sweaty. It is impossible to get a blood pressure in the right arm; in the left it is 130/75. Pulse (apex) is 60 beats/min, regular. The right brachial and carotid pulses are impalpable; left brachial, carotid and both femoral pulses can be felt. There is a grade 2/4 early diastolic murmur at the left sternal edge. He has long fingers and a high arched palate.

QUESTIONS

1. What is the most likely diagnosis and how does it explain the physical signs?

2. What is the differential diagnosis?

3. What complications may occur?

4. What immediate action is indicated?

NOTES FOR REVISION

YOUR ANSWERS

1 Most likely diagnosis and how it explains the physical signs

2 Differential diagnosis

3 Complications that may occur

4 Immediate action indicated

ANSWERS

1. The most likely diagnosis is a dissecting aortic aneurysm, possibly on the basis of Marfan's syndrome (note tall stature, high arched palage, long fingers). The dissection has tracked back to the ascending aorta and destabilized the aortic valve, causing aortic reflux. The intimal flap raised by the dissection has obstructed the brachiocephalic artery, hence the absence of right brachial or carotid pulses. The inappropriate bradycardia may be due to stimulation of aortic arch baroreceptors.

2. Differential diagnoses include pneumothorax, acute myocardial infarction, and ruptured oesophagus; however, none of these will cause this pattern of physical signs.

3. Dissecting aneurysm can cause: death by rupturing into the pleural space of pericardium; stroke by obstructing the cerebral vessels; paraplegia; or renal failure. In addition to Marfan's syndrome, it may be associated with hypertension or other abnormalities of connective tissue.

4. Alert cardiac surgeons cross-match blood. Chest radiography may show widened mediastinum; ECG may show myocardial ischaemia if coronary ostia have been encroached on. Transthoracic echocardiography may show detached aortic valve. CT or MRI scanning provides the most definitive diagnosis.

CASE 19

Fred Park is a 74-year-old retired engineer. At the age of 55 he had an emergency admission to hospital with chest pain, had a cardiac arrest, but was resuscitated. Since then he has taken beta-blockers: at first practolol, and more recently propranolol. He is brought to see you by his daughter, a nurse, who is concerned that her father has become increasingly breathless, and has had to give up his hobby of carpentry. You elicit that Fred now gets breathless on walking about 50 yards, and that on two recent occasions he woke up in the early hours gasping for breath and coughing. On these occasions he brought up white sputum. He denies any chest pain. On systematic enquiry, he says he had jaundice during the war, he smoked until his first hospital admission, and he drinks only on rare social occasions. His current medication consists of propranolol 40 mg bd, a salbutamol inhaler, and ibuprofen for backache.

On examination he was a slim, wiry man. Pulse was 65 beats/min, in atrial fibrillation. JVP was just visible above the clavicle when he sat upright. The cardiac apex was in the 6th left intercostal space in the anterior axillary line. The apex beat was diffuse in character. First and second heart sounds were quiet, and there was a third heart sound. There was a soft, grade 2/6 apical pansystolic murmur radiating to the axillae. The chest was wheezy, but there were also persistent fine basal crepitations (crackles). Abdominal and neurological examination were normal.

QUESTIONS

1. Do you think Fred's breathing problems are due to cardiac or respiratory causes, or both? List the evidence on each side.

2. What is the likely cause of Fred's murmur?

3. How would you alter Fred's medication?

NOTES FOR REVISION

YOUR ANSWERS

1 Cardiac and/or respiratory causes of Fred's problems, and the evidence on each side

2 Likely cause of Fred's murmur

3 How Fred's medication would be altered

ANSWERS 7.38, 7.39

1. Distinguishing between cardiac and respiratory causes of breathlessness is not always easy, especially in the elderly. In Fred's case his wheeze, previous smoking history, dusty hobby and medication with propranolol would all support a 'respiratory' diagnosis. On the other hand, he clearly has heart disease too: he is fibrillating, the JVP is raised, the cardiac apex is displaced and he has basal crepitations in the lungs. His story of waking short of breath would be compatible with paroxysmal nocturnal dyspnoea. The propranolol could contribute to cardiac failure too. On balance, the cardiac evidence is more convincing, but a respiratory contribution cannot be excluded.

2. The murmur is probably due to mitral regurgitation. This could result from mitral ring dilatation secondary to ventricular enlargement, from papillary muscle dysfunction or (unlikely here) from chronic rheumatic disease.

3. Stop the propranolol, treat heart failure with digoxin and an ACE inhibitor, and administer low-dose warfarin to reduce stroke risk from atrial fibrillation.

CASE 20

Philip Simons is a 47-year-old solicitor referred urgently to a hospital outpatient clinic because his wife describes him as waking up gasping for breath at night. Two years ago he had an anterior myocardial infarction, but seemed to make a good recovery. An exercise test at that time showed good exercise tolerance, and a coronary arteriogram at the local BUPA hospital showed only single vessel disease. He was a smoker at the time of his infarct, but has since given up. He denies feeling breathless during the day, but admits to increased tiredness. You are called away from the consultation for a few minutes, and on your return find him not only asleep but snoring!

On examination he weighs 108 kg (244 lb) and has a red face. Pulse is 90 beats/min, regular. Blood pressure is 165/92. There is a suggestion of right ventricular hypertrophy. Heart sounds are normal, the chest is clear, and he can lie flat without distress. JVP is normal; there is no peripheral oedema. The resting 12 lead ECG showed mild right ventricular hypertrophy; the chest X-ray was normal.

QUESTIONS

1. List the arguments for and against a diagnosis of left ventricular failure causing paroxysmal nocturnal dyspnoea.

2. What are the other diagnostic possibilities? Are there diagnostic clues?

3. How could the diagnosis be confirmed?

YOUR ANSWERS

1 Arguments for and against a diagnosis of left ventricular failure causing paroxysmal dyspnoea

2 Other diagnostic possibilities and clues

3 Confirmation of the diagnosis

NOTES FOR REVISION

ANSWERS

1. The arguments for a diagnosis of left ventricular failure causing paroxysmal nocturnal dyspnoea are: the patient's wife is describing paroxysmal breathlessness; the patient has had a known previous infarct; and signs of heart failure might have been masked by diuretic therapy. The arguments against this diagnosis are: such clues as there are point to right rather than left heart failure; there is no orthopnoea; and the chest radiograph does not suggest heart failure.

2. The weight gain, daytime sleepiness and all-day snoring suggest a diagnosis of sleep apnoea syndrome. Episodes of airway obstruction occur during sleep which may be bad enough to cause hypoxia and incipient right heart failure. Daytime sleepiness results from failure to get a proper night's sleep.

3. In this case, sleep studies with videomonitoring and pulse oximetry confirmed severe sleep apnoea. His blood count showed polycythaemia, presumably in response to hypoxia.

CASE 21

Chandika Chauhan is a 19-year-old girl who arrived from Bombay 2 years ago. She complains of feeling generally unwell, of being breathless on exertion and of waking up drenched in sweat. She has had these symptoms for 3 months, but has not complained before because she did not wish to lose time from her university course. Recently, however, she has noticed chest pain which is mainly retrosternal, but occasionally is felt at the tip of her left shoulder. The pain is not related to exertion, but varies with position. She has lost a stone in weight, but thinks this is because of British university food.

On examination, she is in sinus rhythm; her pulse is 100 beats/min, and her blood pressure 100/65. The JVP is raised, and pulsation is easily seen above the clavicle when she is sitting upright. There are some enlarged lymph nodes in the supraclavicular fossae. The cardiac apex is hard to localize. Heart sounds are quiet. A scratchy sound can be heard at the left sternal border when she sits forward and breathes out. The liver is enlarged three fingerbreadths and is slightly tender. There is some ankle oedema. Peripheral pulses are normal.

QUESTIONS

1. What is the likely clinical diagnosis, and the underlying pathological cause?

2. What are the differential diagnoses?

3. What investigations should you do?

NOTES FOR REVISION

YOUR ANSWERS

1 Likely clinical diagnosis and underlying pathological cause

2 Differential diagnoses

3 Investigations to be carried out

ANSWERS

1. The most likely clinical diagnosis is a pericardial effusion. This would explain the raised JVP, the chest pain which varied with position, the quiet heart sounds and poorly localized apex beat, and the scratchy sound would be a pericardial friction rub. The most likely cause in a young person recently arrived from India would be tuberculosis, but systemic lupus erythematosus, lymphoma and chronic renal failure are possibilities. A viral pericarditis would be unlikely with this length of history.

2. The differential diagnoses would need to include a dilated cardiomyopathy, recurrent pulmonary emboli causing right heart failure and chronic rheumatic heart disease.

3. The chest radiograph would show an enlarged cardiac shadow, and might show tuberculous lung lesions. The ECG would show generalized low voltages, and might show 'saddle-shaped' ST-segment elevation. Echocardiograhpy would be the definitive way of showing the effusion. One would expect a raised plasma viscosity and ESR, and perhaps a normocytic anaemia. A Mantoux test with dilute antigen would be helpful, and it might be possible to biopsy one of the lymph nodes. Pericardiocentesis under echoguidance would yield fluid for microscopy and culture.

   Tuberculous pericardial effusions usually have a good prognosis, though a proportion of cases go on to develop chronic constrictive pericarditis.

CASE 22

Karen, a 33-year-old fashion buyer, presents complaining of chest pain. The pain is retrosternal, with some radiation to the left arm and jaw. It characteristically comes on with exertion, and is rapidly relieved by rest. She first noticed it a month ago, and it has progressively worsened with the result that she now has to stop after climbing one flight of stairs. It was particularly bad last week when she had to look for a taxi after a business dinner on a very cold evening. She is a non-smoker, does not take oral contraceptives, and has a 5-year-old daughter.

On examination, Karen's blood pressure was 125/82, pulse 70 beats/min, regular. There was a soft systolic murmur in the aortic area. There was no clinical left ventricular hypertrophy, and the carotid pulse was normal. She had a prominent corneal arcus, there were swellings in the extensor tendons of the hands, and both Achilles tendons were thickened. Her father had died from myocardial infarction at the age of 40, and her elder brother, aged 36, had just undergone coronary bypass grafting. The resting 12 lead ECG was normal.

QUESTIONS

1. On the basis of this information, which is the most accurate of the following statements:
   - Karen has angina
   - Karen has ischaemic heart disease
   - Karen has coronary artery disease
   - It is unlikely that, in a woman of this age, the symptoms have anything to do with the heart.

2. What further questions would you be keen to ask?

3. What is the most likely diagnosis?

4. What further investigations would you do?

5. What advice would you give Karen about her daughter?

NOTES FOR REVISION

YOUR ANSWERS

1 Does Karen has angina, ischaemic heart disease or coronary artery disease? Are these likely in a young woman?

2 Further questions to ask Karen

3 Most likely diagnosis

4 Further investigations

5 Advice to Karen

ANSWERS

1. This is a classic history of angina. Although the symptoms of angina are due to myocardial ischaemia, it is traditional and sensible to use angina to describe the clinical syndrome. It would be wrong to jump to the conclusion that the angina was due to coronary artery disease: it might be due to aortic stenosis or hypertrophic cardiomyopathy. It would be equally wrong to exclude the possibility of angina, despite the rarity of coronary artery disease in women of this age.

2. Angina is uncommon in young women. It would be important to ask about family history (ischaemic heart disease, hypertension, hypertrophic cardiomyopathy); previous rheumatic fever; and murmurs (aortic stenosis). In certain circumstances it might be important to ask about substance abuse (cocaine).

3. The most likely diagnosis is angina due to coronary artery disease resulting from familial hypercholesterolaemia. About one in 500 of the UK population have the heterozygous form of this condition, which usually presents as precocious coronary disease. There are a number of possible gene defects, which lead to phenotypes of differing severity.

4. The most useful tests would be plasma cholesterol estimation and an exercise ECG. Karen's total serum cholesterol was 13.6 mmol/L (normal 3.5–6.4 mmol/L), and her exercise test was strongly positive. Subsequent coronary anteriography showed three vessel disease.

5. There is a chance of 1 in 2 that her daughter will be a heterozygote, and a chance of 1 in 2000 that she will be a homozygote. Referral for cholesterol testing and advice would be appropriate.

CASE 23

Shireen Shams, a 32-year-old florist, feels tired and depressed all the time, and has been suffering from a bout of "flu" which she has not been able to shake off for several months. She has noticed that she has difficulty in getting through the day, particularly as she is on her feet all the time. She aches all over by the evening. After organizing the flowers recently for a wedding she noticed that her fingers were really sore and that there were flecks on her nails. She came to England at the age of 12 and this is the first time she has needed to come to hospital, other than to the dental department to have a wisdom tooth extracted. She had the usual childhood illnesses in Pakistan. On examination she is unwell, with clubbed fingers and an early diastolic murmur. On listening to her heart she explains she has had a "noisy heart" since she was a child.

QUESTIONS

1. What is the likely diagnosis?

2. What physical signs might you elicit?

3. What would be the management?

NOTES FOR REVISION

YOUR ANSWERS

1 Diagnostic

2 Physical signs

3 Management of Shireen's condition

ANSWERS

1. Infective endocarditis.

2. The signs that need to be elicited include fever, splenomegaly and changing murmurs. Endocarditis occurs particularly on valves that have been previously damaged. The patient probably suffered from rheumatic fever in the past. Vasculitis causes splinter haemorrhages in the nails, Osler's nodes (tender nodes in the pulp of the fingers), Roth's spots (haemorrhagic retinal spots) and microscopic haematuria from glomerulonephritis. Large emboli may travel to the brain and result in a stroke.

3. Management should entail: repeated blood cultures to establish an organism and appropriate antibiotics; and antibiotic prophylaxis before any other dental, gynecologic, genitourinary or ear, nose and throat procedure.

CASE 24

Maureen Galloway, a 27-year-old dress-maker, is referred to the gastroenterology department for investigation of an iron deficiency anaemia not responsive to iron tablets. On history she is not vegetarian, has been on oral contraceptives for 7 years with regular periods, takes no other medication, and has not noted any blood in her stool. However, she does complain of diarrhoea, as her motions have changed over the past few years and she now passes four to five large volumes of loose stools daily. In addition, although she eats well, she is losing weight. This does not concern her as she has always considered herself to be overweight. On examination she is pale and her fingers are clubbed. The examiner queries the possibility of splenomegaly. A speck of faeces on the glove after rectal examination is described by the doctor as "typical for steatorrhoea".

QUESTIONS

1. What information should be obtained in a patient with diarrhoea?

2. What clinical findings should be elicited to confirm that a left hypochondrial mass is in fact an enlarged spleen?

3. How might the patient describe steatorrhoeic stool?

4. What diagnosis should be considered in this patient and, if confirmed, would splenomegaly be an unusual finding?

NOTES FOR REVISION

YOUR ANSWERS

1 Information to be obtained in a patient with diarrhoea

2 Clinical findings elicited to confirm an enlarged spleen

3 Description of steatorrhoeic stool by the patient

4 Diagnosis to consider in Maureen. If confirmed, would splenomegaly be an unususal finding?

ANSWERS

8.7, 8.15, 8.29, 8.30

1. The aim is to establish three fundamental facts. First, to establish that the patient actually has diarrhoea. Secondly, to determine whether the diarrhoea originates from the large or small bowel. Thirdly to determine what is the possible aetiology. Diarrhoea by definition is an increase in the volume of stool passed (200–300 g per day). In pseudodiarrhoea frequency is increased, but not volume. In small intestinal diarrhoea pain may occur at any time, and is unrelated to bowel movement. Steatorrhoea is usually indicative of small intestine diarrhoea, whereas the presence of mucus or blood suggests colonic disease. Finally, the diarrhoea which wakes the patient indicates organic pathology, and diarrhoea which resolves with fasting suggests an osmotic aetiology (malabsorption, maldigestion).

2. On palpation an enlarged spleen moves with inspiration, has a notch and enlarges towards the umbilicus. There is no access to the superior surface. On percussion, there is dullness in Traub's space.

3. Steatorrhoeic stool is described as pale coloured, frothy, bulky, extremely smelly and difficult to flush away.

4. Coeliac disease. An enlarged spleen would be unexpected, as the spleen is usually hypoplastic.

CASE 25

Emmanual Cacchacaria, a 65-year-old olive oil importer, complains vociferously of having felt unwell for the past few months, and of being unable to work a full day. He thought this may be due to overwork, but became more concerned when, during the last week or two, he could not fit into his hand-made shoes. The final straw comes when he thinks he is jaundiced. He has no relevant past history, other than an operation for a gunshot wound 30 years earlier, when he had received a transfusion. He does not smoke or drink and takes no medication. On examination, he is jaundiced, has temporal wasting and has bilateral lower limb oedema extending above the knees. He has an enlarged, irregular liver with a bruit. There is no ascites. There are distended veins over the abdominal wall.

QUESTIONS

1. Where is jaundice best observed, and what else causes yellow discoloration of the skin?

2. What causes bruits over the liver?

3. Discuss the possible causes of distended veins over the abdominal wall, and how the flow pattern differs.

4. What is a possible diagnosis in this patient?

NOTES FOR REVISION

YOUR ANSWERS

1 Site where jaundice is best observed, and other causes of yellow discoloration of the skin

2 Causes of bruits over the liver

3 Possible causes of distended veins over the abdominal wall, and how the flow pattern differs

4 Possible diagnosis in Mr Cacchacaria

ANSWERS

8.22, 8.23, 8.28, 8.35, 4.6

1. Jaundice is best observed in the sclera of the eye. The sclera is rich in elastin, for which bilirubin has an affinity. Carotenaemia causes yellow discoloration of the skin, most markedly of the soles, palms, and behind the ears, but not of the sclera.

2. There are two important causes: acute alcoholic hepatitis and hepatocellular carcinoma. Secondary carcinoma of the liver is not associated with a bruit.

3. Distended abdominal veins may be due either to portal hypertension or to obstruction of the inferior vena cava. In the former, the veins radiate from the umbilicus and blood flows away from the umbilicus. In the latter, the veins course up the abdominal wall, with blood flowing towards the heart.

4. The patient has transfusion-acquired hepatitis C, with cirrhosis, and has liver decompensation due to the development of a hepatocellular carcinoma. Extension of the cancer to the inferior vena cava has produced obstruction to this vein.

CASE 26

Horace Salmon, a 79-year-old retired politician, is brought to the emergency room by his wife. She had returned home from her weekly game of bridge to find her husband, a normally fastidious man, still dressed in his pyjamas, with food stains down the front of his top, and urine stains on his trousers. He does not recognize her, and appears lost. She reports that "he has not been himself" for the past few days. She is unaware of any past medical history of note, except possible prostate troubles (he always spends a long time passing urine). However, they never discuss "personal problems". On examination the patient is disorientated for time, place and person, but has no localizing neurological signs. On abdominal examination, he has a pulsatile epigastric mass and there is dullness and percussion from below the umbilicus to the suprapubic region. Rectal examination is performed.

QUESTIONS

1. What are the two main causes of pulsatile epigastric masses, and how can these be distinguished on examination?

2. What is the technique of percussion, and what structure has been percussed in this patient?

3. What does the normal prostate feel like, and what abnormalities may be found in this patient?

4. What is a possible diagnosis?

NOTES FOR REVISION

YOUR ANSWERS

1 The two main causes of pulsatile epigastric masses, and how these can be distinguished on examination

2 Technique of percussion, and the structure percussed in Horace

3 What the normal prostate feels like, and abnormalities that may be found in Horace

4 Possible diagnosis

ANSWERS

3.16, 6.27–6.28, 8.24, 8.25, 8.38–8.39

1. A pulsatile epigastric structure may either be the aorta (normal size, palpated in a thin person, or aneurysmal) or be a mass overlying the aorta (pancreatic or gastric neoplasm). The direction of pulsation indicates whether it arises directly from the aorta (expansile) or from an overlying mass

2. The percussed finger must lie flat on the body surface, parallel to the expected line of dullness. The striking movement must be made with a flick of a wrist, and the percussing finger removed immediately. Percussion should be light over the liver to avoid inflicting pain on the patient.
   The bladder was percussed, indicating urinary retention.

3. The normal prostate has a median sulcus separating the two lateral lobes; the gland measures approximately 3.5 cm in diameter and bulges 1 cm into the rectum. It has a rubbery, smooth consistency. Two possible abnormalities in this patient are benign prostatic hypertrophy (smooth, symmetrical enlargement) and prostatic cancer (asymmetrical, irregular and stony hard).

4. The patient has either benign prostatic hypertrophy or prostatic cancer, leading to urinary retention. The elderly are vulnerable, and the confusion may be due either to this alone, or a superimposed urinary tract infection. In addition, hypercalcaemia should be excluded if cancer is suspected, and chronic renal failure due to obstructive uropathy should be considered.

CASE 27

Ronald Slattery, a 45-year-old salesman, is admitted to the emergency department. He was enjoying a home video when he suddenly felt nauseated, and vomited up a small amount of bright red blood. He returned to the living room, "looking extremely pale" (according to his wife) promptly vomited up a further large quantity of blood and collapsed. When seen by the emergency services he mentions that he has passed black stool for the past few days. Other than a weight gain (his wife describes it as a "beer belly") he has no other medical history. He is on no medications. On examination he has palmar erythema, six spider naevi over his upper chest and neck, and gynaecomastia. The emergency physician elicits signs of ascites and confirms the presence of melena.

QUESTIONS

1. What are the four most common causes of upper gastrointestinal bleeding?

2. How is melena formed, and how is its presence confirmed?

3. What other abnormal signs might be noted on examination of the hands of this patient?

4. What are the physical signs of ascites?

5. What is the most likely diagnosis?

NOTES FOR REVISION

YOUR ANSWERS

1 The four most common causes of upper gastrointestinal bleeding

2 How melena is formed, and confirmation of its presence

3 Other abnormal signs noted on examination of Ronald's hands

4 Physical signs of ascites

5 Most likely diagnosis

ANSWERS

8.10, 8.16, 8.17, 8.21, 8.22, 8.28, 8.29, 8.33

1. Gastric ulcers (30%), duodenal ulcers (21%), gastritis/gastric erosions (9%) and oesophagitis/oesophageal ulcers (8%).

2. In upper gastrointestinal bleeding the blood is denatured by gastric acid and enzymes to hematin. This results in melena (the passage of stools made black and tarry by the presence of altered blood). For practical purposes melena implies bleeding proximal to the ligament of Treitz (the duodenal jejunal junction). Melena must be confirmed by rectal examination since the patient's history of 'dark stool' is notoriously unreliable.

3. If the patient stretches out both arms and hyperextends the wrists with the fingers held separated, a coarse, involuntary flap occurs at the wrist and metacarpophalangeal joints.

4. On inspection the abdominal distension due to ascites is generalized, symmetric and, because it gravitates towards the flanks, may cause the loins to bulge. The umbilicus may become everted. On percussion, there are two characteristic features. First, a gas–fluid interface, and second a change in the position of the gas–fluid interface shown by a change in the patient's position (shifting dullness).

5. The patient has alcohol-induced cirrhosis, with decompensation (as evidenced by the ascites) and a variceal bleed. The oesophageal varices have developed secondary to portal hypertension.

CASE 28

Stella Ziegbrau, an overweight, blonde-haired lady, refers herself to the local emergency department. The previous night she celebrated her 40th birthday, and had prepared a meal for a few of her close friends. The following afternoon she developed epigastric pain, which became progressively more severe over a few hours. She says the pain is constant, and that she "just cannot get comfortable". She is irritated and surprised by the pain as she had not over-indulged in alcohol, and none of her friends has fallen ill. On examination she is apyrexial, and acutely tender in the epigastrium. Her chest X-ray is normal, and an ultrasound scan is scheduled. She is admitted to hospital and given analgesia; however, over the following 24 hours her pain progresses, her vomiting persists, and the ward charts document that she has passed 460 ml urine since admission. On re-examination she is unwell, diffusely tender over the abdomen, and has a bluish discoloration in the flanks.

QUESTIONS

1. What three surgical emergencies should be considered in this patient on presentation, and how does the history differ in these conditions?

2. Is the patient's urine output satisfactory? What causes should be considered in any patient with poor urine output?

3. What clinical sign was found on re-examination?

4. What is the diagnosis in this patient?

NOTES FOR REVISION

YOUR ANSWERS

1 Three surgical emergencies to consider on Stella's presentation, and how the history differs in these conditions

2 Is Stella's urine output satisfactory? What are the causes of any patient's poor urine output?

3 Clinical sign found on re-examination

4 Diagnosis in Stella

ANSWERS

1. Acute pancreatitis, acute cholecystitis and a perforated peptic ulcer. Although a good history is helpful, it is not always possible to differentiate between these three on history. The pain in acute pancreatitis is usually localized to the epigastrium, radiates to the back, is severe and constant, may be partly relieved by sitting forward, and is associated with nausea and vomiting. In acute cholecystitis the pain is often localized to the right hypochondrium, may radiate to the right shoulder, is initially colicky and later becomes continuous. The pain of a perforated ulcer is sudden in onset, intensely severe later, and may radiate diffusely.

2. No. By definition the patient is oliguric (< 400 ml urine in 24 hours). In acute oliguric states consider three possible causes. The tubules may be normal but the glomerular filtration rate is reduced in response to a sodium-conserving stimulus (severe dehydration, systemic hypotension secondary to bleeds, cardiac failure, sepsis). The tubules may be damaged (acute renal failure secondary to acute tubular necrosis, nephrotoxic agents, glomerulonephritis). Finally, there may be outlet obstruction.

3. Grey Turner's sign is caused by seepage of blood stained ascitic fluid along fascial planes to subcutaneous tissues of the loins.

4. Acute haemorrhagic pancreatitis.

CASE 29

Sarah Weston, a 19-year-old high-school student, makes an appointment to see her family doctor. She is extremely anxious. A few months earlier, her mother, then aged 53, had died from metastatic breast cancer. Although deeply upset by this tragedy, Sarah had returned to school and was seemingly coping well. However, last week she read an article in a women's magazine which expanded on the familial risks of breast cancer, and strongly advised regular self examination of the breast. Sarah did this, and was horrified to find what she felt were lumps in her breasts.

QUESTIONS

1. What further information should be obtained on history?

2. What should be looked for on inspection of the breast ?

3. Describe the lymphatic drainage of the breast.

NOTES FOR REVISION

YOUR ANSWERS

1 Further information to be obtained on history

2 What to be looked for on inspection of the breast

3 Lymphatic drainage of the breast

ANSWERS

1. The further history should attempt to determine whether the lumps are benign or malignant. Thus, further questioning needs to establish whether the lump is single or multiple, or unilateral or bilateral. In which quadrant(s) are the lumps, and are the lumps painful? Do the lumps vary in size and tenderness with the menstrual cycle? Has there been any trauma to the breast (although in reality fat necrosis is a rare cause of a hard breast lump, and should be diagnosed only with extreme caution)? Is there any associated nipple tenderness or pain, is there any nipple discharge, and in particular is there a bloody discharge? Finally enquire about the use of the contraceptive pill, and the possibility of pregnancy.

2. The patient must undress to the waist, and sit in front of the examiner. The size and symmetry of the breasts must be noted. The nipples should be observed for symmetry. The skin should be carefully observed for evidence of retraction, dimpling, or peau d'orange. Their presence suggests an underlying malignancy. Manoeuvres to accentuate the presence of tethering should be performed (elevating the arms and pressing the hands against the hips).

3. The medial half of the breast drains to the internal mammary nodes, which are inaccessible for the purposes of examination. The lateral half drains to the ipsilateral axilla, which has five groups of nodes.

CASE 30

Shelley McDonald, a 36-year-old married woman, is woken in the early hours of the morning with pain in the right lower abdomen. The pain is severe (she describes it as being "worse than labour"), constant, worse with movement and associated with nausea. She has vomited once. She is 20 weeks' pregnant. She underwent an amniocentesis at 16 weeks, which was reported as normal. The scan at that stage was also reported as being normal. She has one child, aged 3 years, and has suffered one miscarriage. There has been no vaginal bleeding with this pain, and she describes the pain as different from the miscarriage. On examination she has normal temperature and blood pressure but her pulse rate is rapid. She is exquisitely tender over the right iliac fossa, and lateral to the pregnant uterus there is an ill-defined fullness.

QUESTIONS

1. What would you expect the height of the fundus to be at 20 weeks of pregnancy?

2. What changes are observed on examination of the cervix and vagina?

3. How are the adnexa uteri palpated, and what might be found on examination of the adnexa in this patient?

NOTES FOR REVISION

YOUR ANSWERS

1 Expected height of the fundus at 20 weeks of pregnancy

2 Changes observed on examination of the cervix and vagina

3 Palpation of the adnexa uteri, and what might be found on examination of Shelley

ANSWERS

1. The maturity of the pregnancy can be assessed by examining the height of the fundus. At 20 weeks the fundus should be at the lower border of the umbilicus.

2. In pregnancy the cervix softens (Hegar's sign). The pregnant cervix is said to feel similar to the lip on palpation, whereas the non-pregnant cervix feels like the tip of the nose. In early pregnancy the cervix has a bluish colour due to increased vascularity (Chadwick's sign). The external os of the uterus will be slit shaped or stellate after childbirth. After the birth of a child the pelvic floor muscles may be lax, and on examination of the vagina either a cystocele or a rectocele may be noted.

3. The adnexa are palpated using the bimanual technique. The fingers of the abdominal hand are placed over the iliac fossa whilst moving the vaginal fingers into the lateral fornices, and rotating the finger tips to face the abdominal fingers. The adnexal structures can be felt between the fingertips. In this patient the history and examination findings are suggestive of a torsion of an ovarian (corpus luteal) cyst.

CASE 31

Diana White, a 34-year-old journalist, has just recovered from a urinary tract infection. She returns to her doctor complaining of an intense irritation and itching in the groin region, accompanied by a creamy vaginal discharge.

QUESTIONS

1. Are the itching and discharge a common consequence of urinary tract infection?

2. What additional information would you try to elicit from the history?

3. Give the possible causes of the discharge, indicating the most likely.

YOUR ANSWERS

1 Are the itching and discharge a common consequence of urinary tract infection?

2 Additional information

3 Possible and most likely causes of the discharge

CASE 32

Cindy Tillson, a 26-year-old woman, has just given birth to her first baby, Jake. She complains that her life has changed since giving birth. Most of the day she dashes about between nappy changes, feeds, breast feeding workshops and trying to catch up on her sleep. She feels permanently exhausted. She has noted vaginal bleeding after intercourse. Initially she thought that the bleeding was caused by irregular periods following pregnancy, but now she is seeking advice.

QUESTIONS

1. What examination is essential in this patient?

2. Give the likely causes of the vaginal bleeding.

3. How does the cervix differ before and after pregnancy?

YOUR ANSWERS

1 Essential examination in Cindy

2 Likely causes of the vaginal bleeding

3 Differentiation of the cervix before and after pregnancy

4.9, 9.17–9.19

ANSWERS TO CASE 31

1. The complication is not caused by the urinary infection but is a common result of antibiotic treatment of vaginal infection.

2. Has the patient received broad-spectrum antibiotics? How profuse is the discharge? Does she require protective padding or does she just stain her underwear? Is there a noticeable odour? Has there been abdominal pain or fever? Has the patient had unprotected sex?

3. The possible causes are vaginal infections (candidiasis, trichomoniasis, gardnerelliasis, infection resulting from a retained tampon) and cervical causes (gonorrhoea, herpetic infection and cervical cancer).

   The most likely cause of the vaginal discharge is candidiasis, which is characterized by a creamy white discharge and itching. Vaginal candidiasis often follows a course of broad-spectrum antibiotics.

ANSWERS TO CASE 32

9.24–9.27

1. A cervical examination with a speculum, including a cervical smear and culture.

2. The likely causes are: cervicitis (an inflamed, red cervix and discharge); cervical ectropion (pouting endocervical mucosa following pregnancy); cervical polyps (cherry-red friable polyps arising from the cervix); and cervical carcinoma.

3. Before pregnancy the cervical os is round. During pregnancy, vascularity increases, resulting in a bluish colour (Chadwick's sign). After pregnancy the os is stellate or slit-like.

■ THE MALE GENITALIA

CASE 33

Jonathan Ward, aged 32 years, has returned from a 2-week sports tour in South Africa, accompanied by 16 team-mates. While on tour, Jonathan suffered sunburn and diarrhoea, but was otherwise well. Returning from the airport he complains of aching legs, but receives little sympathy from his wife, who recognizes from his red eyes that he has probably been over-indulging in alcohol. Once home, Jonathan complains of jet-lag and collapses into bed. The next morning he surprises his wife by disappearing early to work. In fact, he visits the genitourinary clinic of the local hospital complaining of burning on micturition and a penile discharge.

QUESTIONS

1. What questions would you want to ask Jonathan whilst taking a history?

2. Give the possible causes of the urethral discharge, indicating the most likely.

YOUR ANSWERS

1 Questions to ask Jonathan whilst taking a history

2 Possible and most likely causes of the discharge

CASE 34

Ross Peterson is seeking advice as he and his wife, Jane, have been experiencing problems conceiving a child. She already has one child from a previous marriage, but the couple have now been trying to conceive for about a year, and Ross is becoming increasingly anxious that he may be infertile. He is desperate not to transmit his fear to Jane. His other medical problem, ulcerative colitis, is usually well controlled, but in recent months has become troublesome, and flared up with all the worry.

QUESTIONS

1. What questions would you particularly like to ask Ross?

2. Which drugs may cause impotence?

3. What do you think may be the cause of Ross's infertility?

YOUR ANSWERS

1 Questions to ask Ross

2 Drugs causing impotence

3 Cause of Ross's infertility

ANSWERS TO CASE 33

10.5, 10.6

1. Venereal disease is a common cause of urethral discharge, and patients concerned about sexually transmitted disease will usually mention the fear of the disease. If this information is not forthcoming, ask the patient directly:
   - Whilst on tour, did you have any unprotected sexual contact?
   - If so, when?
   - Does your partner have any genital disease?

2. These are: gonococcal urethritis; non-gonococcal urethritis; *Chlamydia trachomatis*; *Trichomonas vaginalis*; candida; non-specific urethritis; and Reiter's syndrome.
   Reiter's syndrome. The urethral discharge and dysuria usually occur approximately 2 weeks after diarrhoeal illness (typically Shigella, Campylobacter or Salmonella). The syndrome is usually associated with conjunctivitis (occasionally unilateral) and a seronegative large joint asymmetrical arthropathy. Less commonly there may be circinate balanitis, tendonitis (especially Achilles tendonitis), plantar fasciitis and keratoderma blennorrhagicum, a pustular, scaly rash over the soles of the feet.

ANSWERS TO CASE 34

10.6, 10.7

1. The questions to be asked are:
   - Do you have difficulty obtaining or maintaining an erection?
   - Do you ejaculate?
   - Do you know when Jane ovulates?
   - Are you on any medication or had any cancer treatment?
   - Has there been any change in facial hair growth?

2. These are:
   - Major tranquillizers (e.g. phenothiazines)
   - Lithium
   - Sedatives (barbiturates, benzodiazepines)
   - Anti-hypertensives (methyldopa, debrisoquine, clonidine)
   - Oestrogens
   Alcohol and drug abuse (heroin, methadone) may also cause impotence.

3. Ross may be taking sulphasalazine for his colitis. This causes reversible oligospermia. He should be advised to change his colitis treatment to 5-aminosalicylic acid.

CASE 35

Robert Tobias, a 22-year-old student, has just landed the lead role in the faculty theatre production. He is doubly thrilled because Vanessa, whom he has long admired from afar, is also in the cast. His happiness is only spoilt by one thing: he has noticed a large swelling in the left side of his scrotum. He hoped it would disappear, but instead it appears to be enlarging, causing him considerable concern. He now finds he is constantly worrying about it and summons up the courage to see the campus doctor. On examination it is possible to 'get above' the mass.

QUESTIONS

1. What diagnosis was immediately excluded by the campus doctor?

2. What are the possible diagnoses of the scrotal swelling?

3. How would you differentiate the above by examination?

YOUR ANSWERS

1 Diagnosis excluded by the campus doctor

2 Diagnoses of the scrotal swelling

3 Differentiation of the above diagnoses by examination

CASE 36

Lucien Barker, aged 27 years, has just returned from working as an engineer in Saudi Arabia for the past 2 years. He had a fabulous 'welcome home' party on Saturday night, organized by his brother. Since then, however, he has had an intense burning sensation in the thighs, groin and genitals. Today, Wednesday, he has developed painless lesions on his penis. About 2 months ago, while still in Saudi Arabia, he had a similar problem with penile lesions but the lesions disappeared. The lesions occurred after a rather drunken party to celebrate the end of a project.

QUESTIONS

1. What aspects of the history are you particularly interested in?

2. What is the most likely cause of the lesions?

3. What complications may occur and what is the natural history of this illness?

YOUR ANSWERS

1 Aspects of the history of particular interest

2 Most likely cause

3 Possible complications and history of the illness

ANSWERS TO CASE 35

10.10–10.12

1. Indirect inguinal hernia can be immediately discounted. The swelling arises from the scrotal contents as it is possible to 'get above' the swelling. It is not possible to define an upper margin to an indirect inguinal hernia, which has migrated into the scrotum.

2. The possible diagnoses in Robert are: hydrocele (entrapment of fluid in the tunica vaginalis); an accumulation of fluid in an epididymal cyst; varicocele (varicosity of the veins of the pampiniform plexus); and testicular mass (e.g. carcinoma).

3. It is important to determine whether the swelling is solid or cystic. Cystic swellings are fluctuant and can be transilluminated. A hydrocele is cystic and cannot be separated from the testicle, as it surrounds the organ. An epididymal cyst lies above and behind the testis and can therefore be distinguished from the testis. A varicocele is usually left sided and has the consistency of a ' bag of worms'. If the patient coughs, the impulse can be felt to be transmitted to the varicocele. The varicocele is caused by dilatation of the veins on the pampiniform plexus, is separated from the testis and empties when the patient lies flat. A carcinoma is usually hard and craggy and may be felt as a discrete mass within the testis, or a mass replacing the testicle.

ANSWERS TO CASE 36

10.8–10.9

1. You should clarify whether or not any sexual encounters have taken place, both recently and before the previous episode of penile sores. You should check if a diagnosis was made after the previous episode.

2. Genital herpes. The ulcers seem to be recurrent and he has pain corresponding to the S1–S5 dermatomes. Genital herpes is caused by *Herpes simplex* virus type 2 which causes an initial attack and then lies dormant in the presacral ganglia. Recurrent attacks occur and may have prodromal symptoms of a burning or prickling sensation in the S1–S5 dermatomes (i.e. groin, thigh and genital area). The genital ulcers are initially painless and vesicular.

3. The vesicles may rupture causing painful erosions with a surrounding halo. The erosions may coalesce to form ulcers which can become secondarily infected. The urinary meatus may be affected, causing dysuria. The infection is transmissible and the natural history is for the lesions to spontaneously regress and recur over time.

CASE 37

Tom Carlson, a 7-year-old boy, has just been to his friend Jerry's birthday party. They were going to a nearby hamburger restaurant for the party, but the trip was cancelled as Sarah, Jerry's sister, has mumps. Jerry has vowed never to forgive Sarah for ruining his birthday, although all his friends appeared to enjoy themselves. He has been particularly appeased by a long afternoon of various party games. Later that evening, Tom suddenly feels very unwell and has severe scrotal and lower abdominal pain, so much so that he will not let anyone touch the area. He thinks he may have been hit in the groin during the party.

QUESTIONS

1. What are the possible diagnoses?

2. What would you look for on examination to differentiate the above?

3. What is the treatment for the most likely diagnosis?

NOTES FOR REVISION

YOUR ANSWERS

1 Possible diagnosis

2 What to look for on examination to differentiate the above diagnosis

3 Treatment for the most likely diagnosis

ANSWERS

1. The possible diagnoses are: trauma; torsion; and orchitis.

2. Traumatic testicular pain is unlikely as the pain would occur immediately, not several hours later. In torsion the scrotal skin is reddened and the affected testis lies higher. The testis is exquisitely tender. In orchitis (e.g. mumps) parotitis usually precedes the orchitis and occurs 14 to 18 days after the infection. The testicle is swollen and oedematous, and the patient is generally very unwell, with pyrexia and backache. Mumps orchitis is rare before puberty.

3. Torsion is the most likely diagnosis. This is an emergency requiring surgery to untwist the spermatic cord and fix the testicle within the scrotum.

CASE 38

Sam and Karen Rothman have moved into their new home and spent the whole weekend moving furniture. Sam, aged 35 years, has "put his back out" by trying to shift their double bed, and on Monday morning sees his doctor because he feels unable to work. He works as a caretaker and maintenance manager in a block of residential apartments. Because he has only recently moved to the area, the doctor has never met him before, so Sam explains that he has experienced problems with low-back pain for some time, but never as severe as this.

QUESTIONS

1. What questions would you want to ask Sam?

2. How would you examine him?

3. What may be causing the backache?

4. If, on examination, an ankle reflex could not be obtained, what else would you particularly examine for?

NOTES FOR REVISION

YOUR ANSWERS

1 Questions to ask Sam

2 Examination of the patient

3 Possible cause of the backache

4 What to examine for if an ankle reflex could not be obtained on examination

ANSWERS

1. The questions to be asked are:
   - Does his pain move to his legs?
   - Is this his usual low back pain, or is this something new?
   - Did it start suddenly or come on gradually?
   - Is the pain exacerbated by coughing or leaning forward?

2. The lumbar spine should be tested for tenderness. The range of movements needs to be assessed. Flexion – ask him to touch his toes. Extension and lateral flexion – ask him to slide his arms down the side of his legs, one at a time. The nerve stretch tests need to be carried out: straight leg raising for Bragard's and Lasègue's signs, and femoral stretch test. If straight leg raising is limited by pain to < 45°, the possibility of a lumbar disc prolapse should be considered. A full neurological examination should be performed.

3. His pain may be caused by: musculoskeletal strain – possibly secondary to moving furniture; degeneration of an intervertebral disc – a prolapsed disc can occur, most commonly at L4/5 or L5/S1; spondylolisthesis; osteoarthritis – 'wear and tear' of his lumbar joints resulting in chronic back pain; or ankylosing spondylitis – this condition usually affects male patients, involving first the sacroiliac joints and progressing to involve the spine. The associated stiffness is characteristically relieved by exercise.

4. The ankle jerk is innervated by S1 and sensory changes should be sought in the distribution of S1 (lateral aspect of foot and posterior calf).

CASE 39

Norma Terlington, aged 55 years, has recently become a grandmother and has spent the weekend looking after her daughter, Cherie, and grandson, Bruce. Cherie has found the weekend quite stressful and is rather hoping that her mother is not going to stay much longer. Firstly, her mother's cooking has been somewhat haphazard and she has also been dropping things. Cherie is not too concerned about losing the china poodles, but she hopes that Bruce doesn't get the same treatment. Furthermore, Norma keeps on shaking her right hand as if to try to make it more useful: she says it helps to get rid of the tingling. She omits to tell Cherie that the problem is worse at night, when she is sometimes woken by a pain in her hand.

QUESTIONS

1. How would you examine Norma's hands for weakness?

2. What do you think may be the problem with Norma's right hand, and how would you test for this?

3. Give likely causes of this condition

NOTES FOR REVISION

YOUR ANSWERS

1 Examination of Norma's hands for weakness

2 Problem with Norma's right hands, and how to test for this

3 Likely causes of Norma's condition

ANSWERS

1. The hands should be inspected for any evidence of muscle wasting. The two hands should be compared to assess whether there is wasting of the relevant thenar eminence. The power should then be assessed, testing the muscles supplied by the ulnar and the median nerves. The ulnar nerve supplies the dorsal interosseous muscles, which can be tested by abducting the fingers against resistance. The abductor pollicis brevis is supplied by the median nerve and can be assessed by lifting the thumb vertically against resistance.

2. Carpal tunnel syndrome. This syndrome is caused by compression of the median nerve at the wrist. There is weakness and sometimes wasting of the muscles supplied by the median nerve. Tapping over the median nerve at the wrist may produce tingling in the hand (Tinel's sign). Prolonged flexion of the wrist may have a similar effect (Phalen's manoeuvre).

3. The carpal tunnel syndrome may be caused by soft tissue swelling at the wrist triggered by conditions such as pregnancy, menopause, rheumatoid arthritis, acromegaly, myxoedema and local trauma. Most commonly, however, the condition is idiopathic.

CASE 40

Lord Myers, or Tony to his friends, aged 32 years, is having a bad day. He considers it unthinkable to get out of bed before 10 am, but today he has been rudely awoken by the screams of Mrs Shen, his home help, who arrives to find that there has been a burglary. He gets out of bed reluctantly to see what is happening, using the side of the bed and the bedside table to hoist himself up. He waddles downstairs to find the police have already arrived. Mrs Shen and the police officer sit down over a cup of tea to take details, but Tony remains standing as he knows how difficult it will be for him to stand up again once he has sat down.

QUESTIONS

1. What questions would you want to ask Tony about his weakness?

2. How would you examine Tony's lower limbs in order to investigate the cause of his weakness?

3. Give common non-musculoskeletal causes of this type of lower-limb weakness.

YOUR ANSWERS

1 Questions to ask Tony

2 Examination of Tony's lower limbs

3 Common non-musculoskeletal causes of Tony's lower-limb weakness

CASE 41

James Jefford, aged 47 years, is president of the local wine tasting society, a lover of antique cars, and has succeeded in making it through to the finals of the 'Which Wine?' tasting competition. As he was concentrating on what he thought was a Sancerre, he suddenly noticed that a pain in his toe, which he had woken up with, was becoming unbearable. He sat down, and pulled off his shoe and sock to reveal a very hot, red toe. His opposing finalist was initially concerned, but then upset when the finals were postponed. His wife remembers that he had experienced this problem before, during the Christmas quiz the previous year, when she had ended up driving James home in his antique car.

QUESTIONS

1. How would you examine James' joints?

2. What diagnoses would you consider?

3. How would you confirm the diagnosis?

YOUR ANSWERS

1 Examination of James' joints

2 Differential diagnosis in James

3 How to confirm the diagnosis

ANSWERS TO CASE 40

11.33, 11.43

1. Do, or did other members of his family have problems with walking or weakness? Does he have any sensory difficulties? Are the symptoms experienced equally on both sides?

2. The lower limbs should be examined to assess whether the weakness is symmetrical and if its distribution is predominantly proximal, as suggested by the history. Trendelenburg's sign is likely to be positive: when the patient stands on either leg the pelvis sinks downwards. You should ask him to stand from a sitting position whilst holding his hands away from the body. When patients are allowed to facilitate standing by the use of their hands, they supply the extra power by hoisting the trunk with the aid of arms and hands. With a proximal myopathy the patient will struggle to rise. Patients classically stand by climbing up their legs using their arms in order to extend the trunk – Gowers' manoeuvre.

3. The causes of a proximal myopathy are: thyrotoxicosis; Cushing's syndrome; and osteomalacia.

ANSWERS TO CASE 41

11.39–11.42

1. The foot joints should be examined for signs of acute arthritis (heat and swelling). Other joints should be inspected, including the hands. Are there joint effusions? Is there tenderness of surrounding structures (e.g. tendons). The range of joint movements needs to be assessed.

2. The differential diagnosis of a single hot, swollen joint is gout or septic arthritis.

3. In addition to acutely painful joints, look for evidence of tophaceous gout, e.g. helix of the ear and fingers. The joint must be aspirated: in gout there will be negatively birefringent crystals seen under polarized light. The aspirate must also be examined for organisms and submitted for culture.

CASE 42

Janice Dryden makes an appointment for her husband to see a neurologist. Dr Dryden is a 76-year-old retired physician, who used to take pride not only in his appearance, but also in his general health. He took great pleasure in woodwork and active interest in the latest offerings of the New England Journal of Medicine. He attributed his good health to never having smoked, and drinking in moderation only. Over the past months, Janice had observed a change. Although he appears physically well, he has lost interest in carpentry, complaining that he "is getting old and clumsy". He has stopped reading medical journals, complaining that they "are all science and no medicine". She seeks an appointment when on the way home one day. Her husband, insisting that he knows the way, drives around for an hour before listening to her directions. On general examination there is food on his tie, and his fly is unzipped. The neurologist completes a meticulous examination of the cranial nerves, cerebellum, extrapyramidal system and peripheral nervous system, finds a positive snout reflex (but nothing else) and says that Dr Dryden is perhaps slowing down a little but generally sound for his age. He suggests that the patient simply take it easy for a while.

QUESTIONS

1. Is there any significance in the patient's dress?

2. What basic aspect of any neurological examination was forgotten, and how is this component quickly assessed?

3. What is the snout reflex?

4. What is apraxia, and is this patient apraxic?

YOUR ANSWERS

1 Significance in the patient's dress

2 Forgotten basic aspect of neurological examination, and how this can be quickly assessed

3 The snout reflex

4 What is apraxia? Is Dr Dryden apraxic?

ANSWERS

12.4, 12.8, 12.9, 12.11–12.12

1. Yes. Deterioration in dress and personal care may indicate higher cortical dysfunction. As a crude approach, leaving open one's fly is an early sign, forgetting to open the fly an advanced sign.

2. An assessment of higher cortical function. This patient clearly has a number of features indicative of early dementia. The mini-mental state examination is a screening test which gives a rapid assessment of higher cortical function. This test evaluates orientation, registration, attention and calculation, recall and language. A maximum score of 30 points can be obtained.

3. The snout reflex is a primitive reflex. The primitive reflexes are 'released' either by focal pathology affecting the frontal lobes (e.g. cerebral tumours) or by diseases diffusely affecting the hemispheres bilaterally, giving as their primary clinical manifestation an impairment in higher cortical function (e.g. Alzheimer's disease). The primitive reflexes which can be tested for are the glabellar tap, the palmomental reflex, the pout and suckling reflexes and the grasp reflex.

4. Apraxia is a disorder of skilled movement, not attributable to weakness, incoordination, sensory loss or failure of comprehension. Without details of an examination of high cortical function, it is impossible to say whether the patient is apraxic. Apraxia is a relatively late feature of Alzheimer's disease.

CASE 43

Amanda Hulkin, a 45-year-old divorcee, is taken to the emergency department by her unemployed partner. She is seen by a first-year resident. She reports that over the course of a few hours, weakness has developed in her legs. She says, in some distress, that she is unable to walk properly, and that she has been incontinent and wet her underclothes. She has no other past medical history. She smokes 20 cigarettes per day, and admits to drinking on a daily basis. In confidence, her partner says that she drinks "more than he is happy with". On examination the doctor finds that tone is decreased in the lower limbs. Power is 3/5 in hip extension and knee flexion bilaterally, 4/5 in dorsiflexion and 3/5 in plantar flexion bilaterally. Reflexes are possibly decreased in the knees bilaterally, and absent in the ankles. Plantars are downgoing. The doctor is busy, but runs his hands over the anterior aspects of the lower limbs and feels that the patient has a stocking distribution sensory loss. Joint position testing is performed for the big toes, and noted to be absent. He diagnoses a probable alcoholic peripheral neuropathy, and discharges Amanda with an appointment to see a neurologist one week later. A few days after, the patient is admitted to another hospital.

QUESTIONS

1. What is the Medical Research Council (MRC) grading of muscle power?

2. What nerve roots subserve the ankle and knee jerks?

3. Does this patient have an upper or lower motor neurone lesion, and what are its features?

4. What was omitted in the examination of this patient's sensory system?

NOTES FOR REVISION

YOUR ANSWERS

1 The MRC grading of muscle power

2 Nerve roots subserving the ankle and knee jerks

3 Does Amanda have upper or lower motor neurone lesion? What are its features?

4 What was omitted in the examination of Amanda's sensory system?

ANSWERS

12.65, 12.68, 12.72, 12.78

1. There are five grades in the MRC classification. Grade 0: total paralysis. Grade 1: flicker of contraction. Grade 2: movement with gravity eliminated. Grade 3: movement against gravity. Grade 4: movement against resistance but incomplete. Grade 5: Normal.

2. The root subserving the deep tendon reflexes of the ankle is S1; those for the knee, L2, 3, 4.

3. The patient has a lower motor neurone lesion. Features of a lower motor neurone lesion are muscle weakness, depressed deep tendon reflexes, fasciculation, wasting and flaccidity.

4. The doctor omitted to examine sensation on the back of the legs, and the saddle area. The sensory dermatomes S1 and S2 extend from the side of the foot up the back of the lower limb. S3, S4 and S5 subserve the saddle region. It is not uncommon that these areas are overlooked in the neurological examination of the lower limb. In one postgraduate examination, only 2 out of 10 candidates asked to examine the lower limbs actually tested for sensory deficits in this area. It is critical to avoid missing a cauda equina lesion, which this patient had.

CASE 44

Song Hai Woo, a 29 year-old-political refugee from China, seeks medical attention. He complains that over the past few months he has had a blocked nose. Sometimes when he blows his nose he notes blood. He also reports a headache, which he finds difficult to localize. Over the past few days he has been coughing whilst swallowing, especially with liquids. On examination the patient appears well nourished. He has a palpable, non-tender mass below the left mandibular angle. On neurological testing, higher cortical function is normal, and cerebellar and peripheral nervous system examinations are also normal. On careful cranial nerve examination the patient is found to have a left sided 9th, 10th and 11th cranial nerve lesion.

QUESTIONS

1. How is the 9th cranial nerve examined?

2. How is the 10th cranial nerve examined?

3. In which condition do supranuclear lesions result in clinically significant lesions of the 9th, 10th and 11th cranial nerves?

4. What is the possible diagnosis?

NOTES FOR REVISION

YOUR ANSWERS

1 Examination of the 9th cranial nerve

2 Examination of the 10th cranial nerve

3 Condition in which supranuclear lesions will result in clinically significant lesions of the 9th, 10th and 11th cranial nerves

4 Possible diagnosis

ANSWERS

12.56, 12.57, 12.58

1. The visceral efferent and afferent fibres of the glossopharyngeal nerve are not readily testable. The 9th nerve is tested by examining the gag reflex. Stimulus is applied to the tonsillar fossa. The sensory afferent arc travels in the glossopharyngeal nerve, and the motor efferent arc is supplied by the vagus, resulting in midline elevation of the palate. In a ninth nerve lesion the sensation will be different or absent on the affected side and the gag reflex absent or depressed when elicited on that side.

2. Spontaneous (during phonation) and reflex (on testing the gag reflex) movements of the uvula are assessed. In a unilateral 10th nerve lesion the soft palate deviates to the intact side (the vagus pulls up the soft palate, thus unilateral lesions cause deviation to the contralateral side; the 12th nerve pushes out the tongue, thus unilateral lesions cause deviation to the ipsilateral side).

3. When the lesions are bilateral, a unilateral interruption of corticobulbar tracts to the nucleus ambiguus (the motor nucleus for the 9th, 10th and 11th nerves) usually is of no clinical significance, as the nucleus ambiguus has dual innervation (i.e. receives input from both ipsilateral and contralateral corticobulbar tracts).

4. A nasopharyngeal tumour with invasion of the jugular foramen.

CASE 45

Oriel Minkop, a 54-year-old housewife, is brought to the emergency department by the ambulance service. She gives the following history. Whilst putting up a hem the fingers of her right hand became clumsy, then weak, and she was unable to continue her work. She attempted to stand, but felt as if her right leg was giving way. She sat down again, and called for her husband. Normally a garrulous person, she could not communicate the problem. He thought she was confused and called the emergency services. During the wait for the ambulance, she felt progressively stronger in the hand and leg, and at the hospital gave a clear history but still stumbles over some words. She smokes 15 cigarettes daily and has no other medical history of note.

QUESTIONS

1. What are the three major types of speech defect?

2. What speech problem did the patient have, and what speech problem might she now have?

3. Given the most likely diagnosis, what aspect of the cranial nerve examination might be particularly helpful?

NOTES FOR REVISION

YOUR ANSWERS

1 The three major types of speech defect

2 Speech problem Oriel had and might now have

3 Aspect of the cranial nerve examination that might be particularly helpful

ANSWERS

12.7, 12.10, 12.27

1. The three speech defects are dysarthria, dysphonia and dysphasia. Dysarthria is a defect of articulation without any disturbance of language function. Dysphonia is a defect of speech volume and dysphasia is a defect of language function, with abnormality of speech comprehension and/or production.

2. The patient had a non-fluent dysphasia, probably a Broca's dysphasia (alternative terminology: motor dysphasia, expressive dysphasia). Her present speech difficulty sounds like anomic aphasia where, as with Broca's dysphasia, comprehension is relatively well preserved but, unlike Broca's dysphasia, speech is fluent and interrupted more by pauses than word substitutions.

3. The visual field assessment. The patient's history is typical of a transient ischaemic attack. The combination of a Broca's dysphasia, and weakness in the right limb and leg localise the lesion to the distribution of the left middle cerebral artery. If there is still evidence of a right homonymous hemianopia it might be inferred that the mainstream of the artery has been affected. If not, then either resolution has occurred or the lesion may have been in the superior trunk.

CASE 46

The medical resident is called to the emergency department to assess a young comatose girl. The distraught mother says that her daughter had been extremely despondent over her exam results, and had locked herself into her room 3 days ago. She became more concerned when, one day ago, she heard her daughter vomiting. On the day of admission her daughter had not responded to any questions, and she called the police. They forced open the door to find the daughter comatose, with vomit-stained bedding, and an empty medication bottle on the dresser. The resident checks her blood glucose level, which is low, and initiates a dextrose infusion. As he walks off he says, somewhat callously "There's not much hope: she's got no doll's eye movements". The intern does a careful neurological examination, including a coma score, noting also that the patient is jaundiced.

QUESTIONS

1. What are 'doll's eye movements', and how are they elicited?

2. What should be noted on examination of the pupils in an unconscious patient?

3. What does the Glasgow coma scale assess?

4. What is a possible diagnosis?

NOTES FOR REVISION

YOUR ANSWERS

1 What 'doll's eye' movements are, and how they are elicited

2 What should be noted on examination of the pupils in an unconscious patient

3 What the Glasgow coma scale assesses

4 Possible diagnosis

ANSWERS

12.33, 12.89, 12.90

1. The doll's head manoeuvre tests the doll's eye or oculocephalic movements. The head is moved from side to side or vertically. If the brainstem is intact this manoeuvre will elicit reflex eye movements in the opposite direction to the movement of the head turning (so as to leave them directed forwards). In the conscious patient, however, such a response will be suppressed by visual fixation mediated by the cerebral hemispheres. Thus if the doll's head manoeuvre in a comatose patient is present, this implies disinhibition of the brainstem reflexes by damaged cerebral hemispheres, but the brainstem is intact. If doll's head movements are absent in a comatose patient, there is either structural damage to the brainstem, or a severe depression of brainstem function by some metabolic process.

2. The pupil symmetry, size and response to light. Pupillary reaction to light and the presence of reflex eye movements are of prognostic importance, with a death rate of up to 95% reported in patients who have lost these 6 hours after onset of coma.

3. The Glasgow coma scale assesses the patient's eye opening (1–4, none scores 1), best verbal response (1–5) and best motor response (1–6). Thus a maximum of 15, and a minimum of 3.

4. A paracetamol (acetaminophen) overdose, the clues being the hypoglycaemia and jaundice, and an interval of perhaps four days after taking the overdose prior to the development of complications.

CASE 47

Cindy Kaye, aged 17 years, is learning to drive. It has not been easy, either for herself, or the instructor. She has her driving test next week and wakes one morning, all set for another day of learning the rules of the road, but she does not feel right: her face hurts and she has been dribbling during the night. Looking in the mirror she has difficulty smiling fully, and cannot insert her right contact lens. A wave of panic comes over her: these are the symptoms that her grandmother suffered from, and she is now living in a home for the elderly, unable to walk. She bursts into tears, and notices to her horror that the tears only come from her left eye.

QUESTIONS

1. Which nerve has been affected?

2. What is the condition called, and give common causes.

3. How would you differentiate this condition from other causes of facial paralysis?

YOUR ANSWERS

1 The affected nerve

2 Cindy's condition and its common causes

3 How to differentiate the condition from other causes of facial paralysis

---

NOTES FOR REVISION

ANSWERS

1. The facial nerve (7th cranial nerve) has been affected.

2. This is a lower motor neurone facial paralysis, and the common causes are: Bell's palsy (idiopathic paralysis); Ramsay–Hunt's syndrome (the consequence of herpes zoster affecting the geniculate ganglion); parotid carcinoma; sarcoidosis; and multiple sclerosis.

3. A lower motor neurone facial palsy affects all the facial muscles equally on the affected side, including the frontalis muscle. Therefore the patient is unable to raise their eyebrow on the affected side, in addition to the problem with the other facial movements. In an upper motor neurone lesion there is again asymmetry of the lower face, but the frontalis muscle has bilateral innervation and therefore is unaffected.

CASE 48

Katie Nelson, a 25-year-old accountant, has just given birth. Towards the end of pregnancy, she felt unsteady but ascribed this to her large size. Her problem began as soon as the epidural anaesthetic wore off and now she keeps falling over. In addition, she has difficulty bottle feeding her baby: her hand trembles excessively. Her husband is in the army, posted overseas. When she phones to tell him that he now has a son, she loses control of the volume of her voice and her speech is slurred. Her husband assumes she is over-emotional. Twenty-four hours later the symptoms still persist.

QUESTIONS

1. What would you be looking for whilst examining Katie's gait?

2. What else would you like to examine in this lady?

3. Give three underlying causes of this condition.

YOUR ANSWERS

1 What to look for whilst examining Katie's gait

2 What else to examine in Katie

3 Three underlying causes of the patient's condition

NOTES FOR REVISION

ANSWERS

11.44–11.45, 12.75–12.76

1. Check first of all that the patient can stand and walk unassisted. Then watch the patient walking in a straight line, turn around and walk back. Check the base of the gait (narrow or wide based?) particularly as she turns to see if she becomes unsteady. She may deviate to one side on walking. If the patient has a subtle gait disturbance, heel-to-toe walking may accentuate any disturbance. Cerebellar lesions result in a wide based gait, particularly with mid-line lesions. There is deviation to one side on walking.

2. Katie has gait ataxia, upper limb tremor and dysarthria, all suggestive of a cerebellar problem. The speech should be assessed for erratic pitch and volume. The upper limb may demonstrate an intention tremor. The finger-nose test may show past pointing. Dysdiadochokinesia can be shown by asking her to alternate pronation and supination of the hand: where there will be fluctuations in the speed and amplitude. The eyes should be examined for nystagmus.

3. Cerebellar disease may be caused by multiple sclerosis, tumours (particularly metastatic deposits), alcoholic damage (particularly causing midline damage) or familial cerebellar atrophies.

CASE 49

Harold Gallo, aged 68 years, lives with his daughter. His wife died 2 years previously and subsequently he became increasingly depressed. He used to be an active member of a local bowls club but stopped playing about a year ago, claiming that he felt unable to control the ball well enough. Now he can be seen sitting, as though watching others play, but in reality he seems mostly to stare into space. His daughter hoped that by his moving in with her he might have become more animated, but he has sunk into progressive apathy, and shuffles around the house. In despair she takes him to a doctor, to see if he needs antidepressants.

QUESTIONS

1. What would you look for on examination?

2. What is the likely underlying pathological problem?

3. What treatment may be of help?

YOUR ANSWERS

1 What to look for on examination

2 Underlying pathological problem

3 Helpful treament for Harold

CASE 50

Sylvia Brass is a 42-year-old voluntary worker in the local hospital. For the past 2 weeks she has noticed a mid-thoracic back pain, worse on coughing. She was helping out at the hospital café when she missed her footing and fell over, knocking over a bottle of ketchup which spilt over her right leg. She stood up to go and wash it off, and again her left leg 'gave way'. She managed to hobble to the washroom to wipe clean her leg. This proved difficult because she could not get the water hot enough. On walking back to the café, she fell over again and had difficulty getting back up, so that, despite her protestations, she is taken to the emergency department. There she recognizes the doctor as Dr Tim, who looked after her when she had her breast operation three years ago. He assumes that she has come about the scald on her right leg, but she admits not to have noticed this and that it is in fact her stiff left leg that's the problem.

QUESTIONS

1. On examination you find her arms are completely normal, but her legs are not. What would you expect to find in the left leg?

2. In view of the history with her right leg, what do you think may be the problem here?

3. What is the most likely cause of the problem?

YOUR ANSWERS

1 What to expect in the left leg

2 Possible problem with the right leg

3 Most likely cause of the problem

ANSWERS TO CASE 49

12.70–12.71, 12.73

1. Harold probably has a Parkinsonian syndrome and therefore tremor, rigidity and bradykinesia should be sought for. The tremor is likely to be present at rest and may be pill-rolling in type. Rigidity in the upper limb is likely to be found at the wrist or elbow. The rigidity is either lead-pipe or cogwheel in character. Bradykinesia produces an expressionless face, a slowing of skilled hand movements (in polishing, for example) and changes in the gait, which becomes hesitant and shuffling (festination).

2. Parkinson's disease is due to degeneration of dopaminergic neurones in the substantia nigra.

3. Treatment is symptomatic with dopaminergic drugs (e.g. levodopa with a dopa-decarboxylase inhibitor, or bromocriptine).

ANSWERS TO CASE 50

12.72, 12.86

1. The left leg is described as "stiffer" and has also "given way". It is therefore weaker, suggesting an upper motor neurone lesion and one would expect there to be increased tone, possibly with clonus. The power will be reduced in the leg, and there will be hyperreflexia.

2. She has scalded her right leg without realizing it. This suggests a loss of pain and temperature sensation in that leg. Her arms are described as normal and so the diagnosis of a unilateral cord lesion, a Brown–Séquard's syndrome, is likely, at the level of the thoracic pain. In a unilateral cord lesion, there is contralateral loss of pain and temperature from a level slightly below that of the lesion. There is an ipsilateral loss of pain and temperature at the lesion. There is an ipsilateral loss of proprioception and paralysis below the lesion.

3. Her previous breast operation and the Brown–Séquard's syndrome suggest the diagnosis of carcinoma of the breast with a secondary deposit affecting the cord. Other causes include trauma and multiple sclerosis.

CASE 51

Matt Stevens, 24 years old, has had a particularly successful day playing rugby. However, his girlfriend Olivia is horrified at his appearance: he has an extensive bruise to the right eye and he has lost two front teeth. She takes him to the local hospital the next morning to see if they can fit him with some temporary teeth, and after it has been explained this cannot be done on a Sunday morning, he is given some written instructions regarding a head injury. Matt is unable to read these owing to double vision and his eyes are examined more fully. His right eye has periorbital swelling and he has difficulty opening the eye. Furthermore the right eye seems to bulge. On attempting to examine the movements the right eye does not seem to move, whilst the left moves fully.

QUESTIONS

1. Which nerves control which extraocular muscles?

2. How would you examine a patient complaining of double vision in order to establish which eye is the cause of the problem?

3. Which nerves are affected, and what is the most likely cause of the problem?

NOTES FOR REVISION

YOUR ANSWERS

1 Nerves controlling extraocular muscles

2 Examination of a patient with double vision to establish which eye is causing the trouble

3 Nerves affected, and most likely cause of this problem

ANSWERS

12.29–12.32, 12.34–12.36, 12.42

1. The 4th cranial (trochlear) nerve supplies the superior oblique muscle which is involved in looking down in adduction. The 6th cranial (abducens) nerve supplies the lateral rectus muscle which is responsible for abduction. The 3rd cranial (oculomotor) nerve supplies the rest of the muscles, the levator palpebrae superioris, and pupillary muscles that cause constriction.

2. First, one eye should be covered to establish that the diplopia resolves – confirming binocular diplopia. Establish which image disappears on covering the eye – the false image from the affected eye is the peripheral image.

3. Matt's right eye does not seem to move. In addition, he has a ptosis and therefore seems to have 3rd, 4th and 6th nerve palsies. These, in the presence of proptosis and after trauma, suggests a cavernous sinus thrombosis.

CASE 52

Dennis Ogden, a 52-year-old bus driver, has been sent to the optician by his wife. She feels that one of his eyes looks a little odd. His annual medical examination is scheduled for next week. It is vital that he passes the exam since redundancies are rumoured and, as it is, his chest seems to play up at the thought of being made to see a doctor. He continuously smokes on the way to the optician in an attempt to calm his chest and nerves. Once he gets to the optician he tries on a number of frames, but, somehow, none of them seems to suit him. His eyes look unequal; in fact his right eye seems to have sunken in below his eyelid. This starts him laughing nervously, which sets his cough off. The receptionist spots him and is unamused to see him coughing his mucky, bloody sputum all over the display frames.

QUESTIONS

1. If you were the doctor conducting the annual medical examination, what would you like to investigate further about his health?

2. If you were the optician, what might you notice about Dennis?

3. At which sites may pathology occur to give this problem?

NOTES FOR REVISION

YOUR ANSWERS

1 Further investigation about Dennis' health by the doctor conducting the annual medical examination

2 What might be noticed about Dennis by his optician

3 Sites at which pathology may occur to give this problem

ANSWERS

6.13–6.14, 6.23, 11.31, 12.36–12.37

1. Dennis has a cough productive of 'mucky, bloody sputum' and he is a smoker. He therefore requires a chest X-ray to look for a possible carcinoma of the bronchus.

2. The optician (and the doctor) will be looking for any difficulty reading road signs, and also checking on his 'unequal eyes'. With his possible carcinoma of the bronchus, a Horner's syndrome should be considered with ptosis being the most obvious sign, and then looking for a narrow palpebral fissure, miosis, anhidrosis and enophthalmos.

3. Horner's syndrome results from interruption of the sympathetic nerve supply to the pupil. It may occur with pathology in the brain stem, cervical cord or thoracic outlet (if due to a carcinoma of the lung, this is Pancoast's syndrome, the commonest cause), or with a carotid artery aneurysm.